FITNESS EQUIPMENT
A Shopper's Guide

How to Research, Evaluate and Purchase the Perfect Exercise Equipment for Your Home Gym

Tim Adams

From the Author

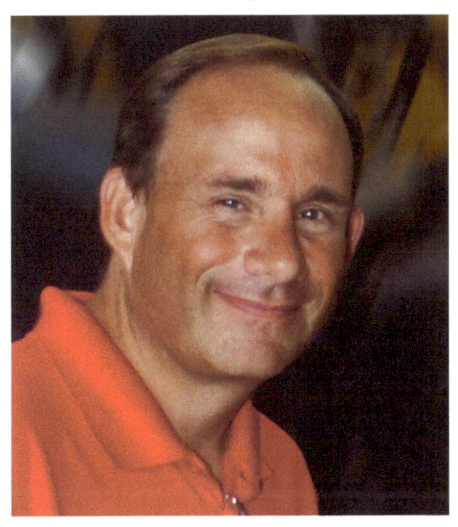

My name is Tim Adams and I own RX Fitness Equipment in Thousand Oaks, California. Thanks for taking the time to look over my book. I've been matching people with the right equipment for their fitness goals and budgets for 30 years, and whether I'm outfitting an entire commercial facility or selling a single treadmill or spin bike, my objective is always the same; to be sure that my customers get what THEY need – not what I would like to sell. This short book is the next logical step toward that objective. I hope it will allow me to reach people that I may never meet face to face, as well as some who might one day come into my store. The better informed my customers are, the better I can serve them. My business is built on developing life-long relationships, not on selling a single piece of equipment that, in three months, will become a clothes rack.

My goal is to help you get fit and stay fit for the rest of your life, not to send you home with an expensive piece of equipment based on a New Year's resolution or because you were briefly feeling bad about yourself. If you buy something from me, whether it's a $4000 treadmill or a $40 kettlebell, I want it to be something you'll use for a long, long time. Figuring out, as best you can, what that is before you buy it is always the preferred way to go. I hope this book helps.

Table of Contents

Introduction

Getting fit is an admirable goal that, once accomplished, is not just a fleeting prize but can be a lifetime triumph. While the thought of getting fit may seem daunting, the payoff is well worth the effort. It's not just about physical changes – it's a lifestyle change that leads to greater happiness and success. You're reading this because you want greater happiness and success, because you want to be the best you that you possibly can be, and because you've decided that you're ready to make the investment in time and action – a decision that will lead to a fitter, healthier you.

While it might strike you as an overwhelming task, getting fit doesn't have to be as hard as it looks. In fact, with just a few lifestyle adjustments and equipped with this guide, you'll be well on your way to a

SportsArt Functional Trainer A93

great payoff. First, trim your diet to incorporate healthier meal choices – more vegetables, fruits, and proteins, and fewer processed foods. Then, develop the right attitude. Your mind can make all the difference between success and failure because it, too, is a muscle which needs to be trained. As they say, getting fit is not a sprint but a marathon. With an improved diet, a dedicated and open mind, and the right equipment, you'll soon find that regular exercise becomes first a routine, then a habit, and then an enjoyable part of your everyday life.

Follow this guide to determine the best fitness equipment for you – equipment that fits your fitness and health goals as well as your budget requirements. With a little planning and consideration, every piece you purchase will be well-suited to your fitness goals without breaking the bank and will be well-loved and well-used. Whether you want a complete home gym or a single piece of equipment, use this guide to learn the differences between types of fitness equipment, what they're used for and how they might benefit you and, most importantly, whether or not they will be a good fit for your specific needs.

We wish you success in your search for the right equipment as well as your quest to be a better, healthier you. We've covered the explanations and details so that you can intelligently narrow down your choices and go shopping without having to rely on the hype of marketing or the opinions of salespeople. By investing a little time up front, you will educate yourself, save money and become a savvy fitness equipment shopper. Read on.

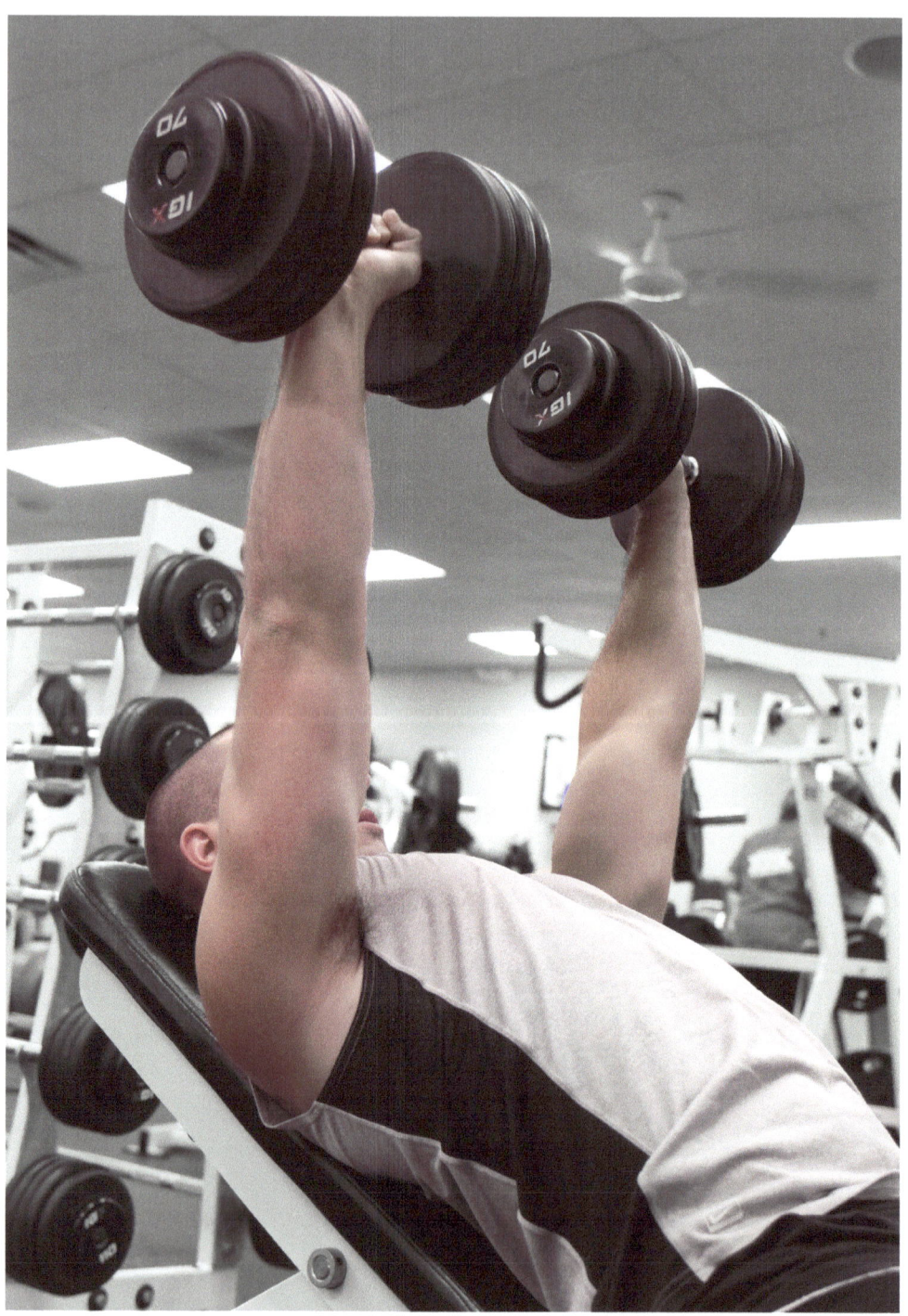

Chapter 1

Assess Your Goals and Needs

Every task benefits from some self-reflection. Before you embark on a fitness equipment quest and shell out thousands of dollars for pieces that might end up gathering dust, set aside some time to ask yourself a few questions first. Bring out a pen and a pad of paper and record your answers.

First, ask yourself what your fitness goals are. Is it simply to lose weight? Gain muscle? Are you trying to trim down to the ultimate runner's body? What are you using your body for? Are you a runner, bodybuilder, swimmer, or just someone who would like to be in better shape? Don't think just in terms of immediate goals — think long-term. Think of the kind of equipment you'll need to not only achieve but to maintain your fitness goals.

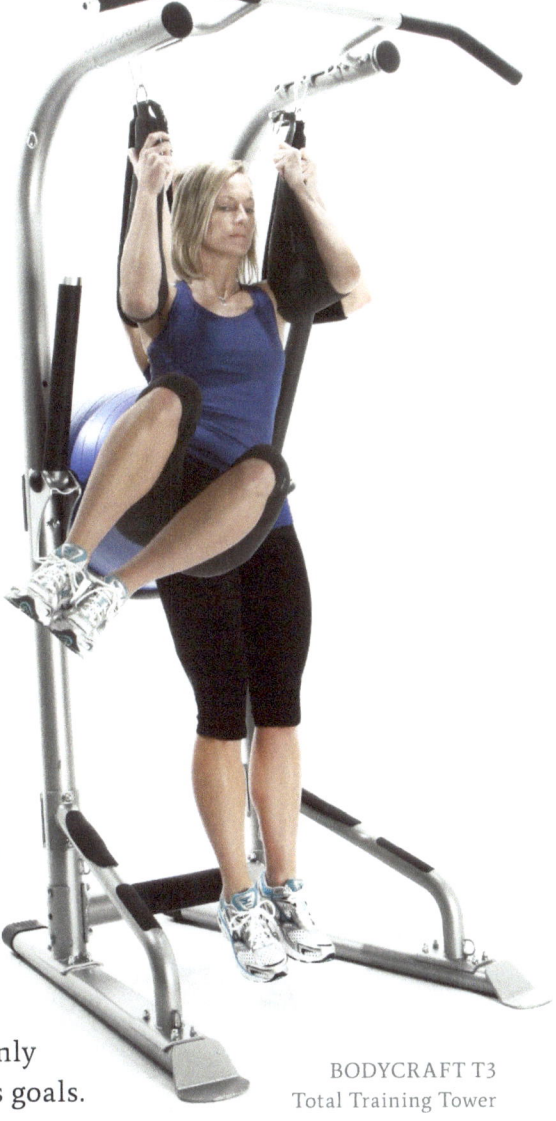

BODYCRAFT T3
Total Training Tower

Create a list of questions and answer them with brutal honesty. How many times a week do you plan on exercising? You might be starting out with a small number, maybe once or twice a week, but after your exercise habits are formed, how many times a week do you expect you'll work out? Are you planning to work out strictly at home or incorporate other types of exercise also? For example, if you're a distance runner and enjoy running outside, perhaps a treadmill wouldn't be as useful as some light weights, which can help tone and work out muscles you don't normally use while running. If you're more focused on cardio, you won't need a lot of weights for that either but will choose exercises and equipment that will raise your heart rate.

Assess your interior space. Where will you be placing your exercise equipment? Have you designated a space for your workouts? Do you have an entire room available, or just one small corner? Is it space in your garage, or in your backyard? Measure the space or spaces you will set aside and see just how much room you have to work with. Be sure to write down your measurements. The less room you have, the more selective you'll have to be in choosing equipment. Depending on your available space, you might have to consider an all-in-one machine over multiple machines. If you only have room outside, you should look at machines made out of the most durable materials possible. If you'll be using inside space, also consider the floor material. Weights, or even a frequently used machine, can damage tile or wood floors and leave marks in the carpet. Consider purchasing interlocking gym floor mats or other resilient flooring for your exercise space.

Keep in mind that atmosphere does matter. Before buying anything, visualize your space. If you're building an entire home gym, you'll ideally have free reign to modify all aspects of it. If you're lucky enough to be able to dedicate a whole room or your garage to your exercise program, you'll be able to fully customize your space, constrained only by budget. If you're not planning on setting up an entire home gym and want only a few pieces of equipment, then adjust your plan accordingly.

Figure out your lighting situation. Would a room without a window be depressing to you, or is it inconsequential? Decide how much and what kind of lighting you'll need as well as the aesthetics of the other surroundings. You may want to paint the walls a different color, change the floor, or install a music system. Putting up posters or other decorations can help motivate you and make the space feel more your own. Write down all the factors you want to consider and then prioritize them. Keep them handy for reference as your plan moves forward.

Finally, look at your finances. How much money are you willing to spend on fitness equipment? Come up with a solid number that will serve as your max budget. You can work and rework your intended purchases within this number, but setting a maximum spend level will keep you anchored and will help you assess your priorities. It will also help ward off buyer's remorse or other regrets. By spending only an amount you've deemed comfortable, you'll invest it much more carefully and vastly increase the chances that you'll actually value and use your exercise equipment regularly. Remember, the objective is to buy useful equipment that will serve your goals and won't end up gathering dust in your garage.

Create a plan. Write down your fitness goals, your space restrictions and your budget. Have these available any time you're making decisions about a purchase or a space modification. Keeping these parameters in mind will allow you to organize your purchases. When looking at equipment, think to yourself, "Okay, I need something that's X" by Y" in size, costs less than $X and fills this role in my fitness plan." That kind of analysis will allow you to quickly pinpoint the best equipment for you in each category.

With your plan in place the first things to look at, when it comes to equipment, are the items that will compose the environment around your fitness equipment. These will become the framework of your exercise room.

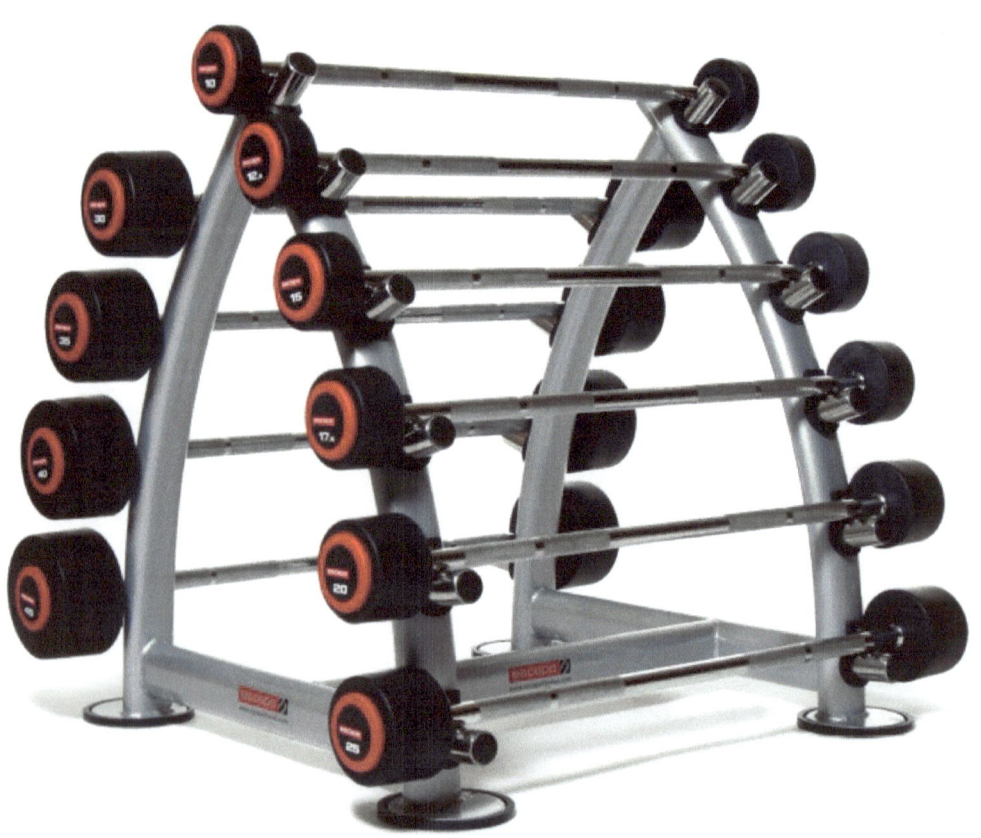

Escape 10kg - 45kg SBX Rubber Barbell Set with Rack

Chapter 2
Setup: Floor Mats, Racks, etc.

It's not just the equipment itself that makes a fitness machine effective. Surroundings matter too. To help you achieve success, your environment should be tailored specifically around exercise.

First, consider the floor. Working out on hardwood and tile floors quickly becomes uncomfortable, especially when doing body weight exercises or stretches. Hard floor surfaces can also be dangerous. If you fall or drop something, you risk not only damaging the floor but hurting

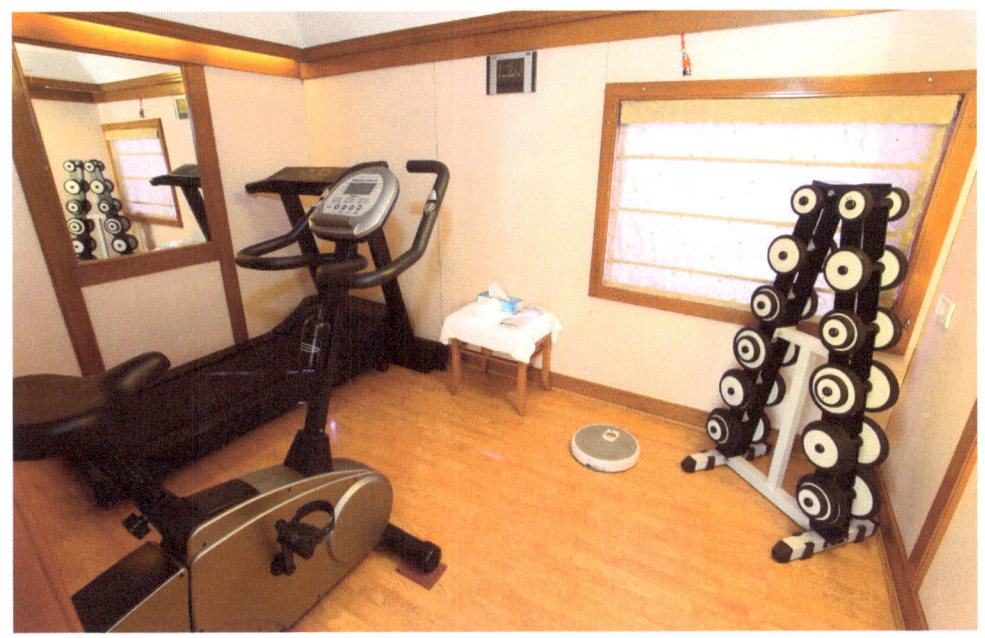

Photo by Simon Pielow

yourself as well. If your budget allows, consider investing in resilient wall-to-wall flooring, such as interlocking gym flooring or floor mats. If that's not practical, individual floor mats come in a variety of colors, sizes, and thicknesses. For standard flooring, get rubber mats that are at least one inch thick. For gym mats, like those you often see in public gyms, get something at least two to three inches thick. These mats will support your back and limbs when you do stretches, yoga and other body exercises as well as activities like jumping rope. You should only need one or two mats a few feet long for all your needs unless you plan to be working out with multiple people, in which case you'll need more mats.

Next, you need to think of storage capacity. You need a system that will allow organization of all your equipment. While machines are freestanding and don't need boxes or cases, things like dumbbells, kettlebells, exercise balls, yoga mats, and similar items can quickly clutter your exercise space. Investing in a few racks to store your supplies is a great idea. Racks come in lots of shapes and sizes, from simple racks to pyramid racks and others. Most racks are rubber, metal, or some combination thereof. Metal racks tend to last longer, but are heavier. They can also rust if left outside. Rubber racks tend to be cheaper, lighter, and more weather-resistant. However, be aware that some rubber racks have one serious, little-known flaw; a pungent odor. For whatever reason, many rubber racks retain an oily scent which cannot be washed away or perfumed over. If you're in a small enclosed space, this smell can quickly taint the air and make working out unpleasant. Some racks with rubber guards may also leave stains on your dumbbells, depending on the composition of your dumbbells. Keep in mind that, regardless of the rack you choose, unless you buy locally it will likely be shipped to you in parts. You will then have to assemble it yourself upon arrival.

You might not want to spend the additional money, but racks are an excellent investment. They will keep your home gym tidy, safe, and will save you many future headaches. Order racks for all your loose items so that your gym stays neat and organized.

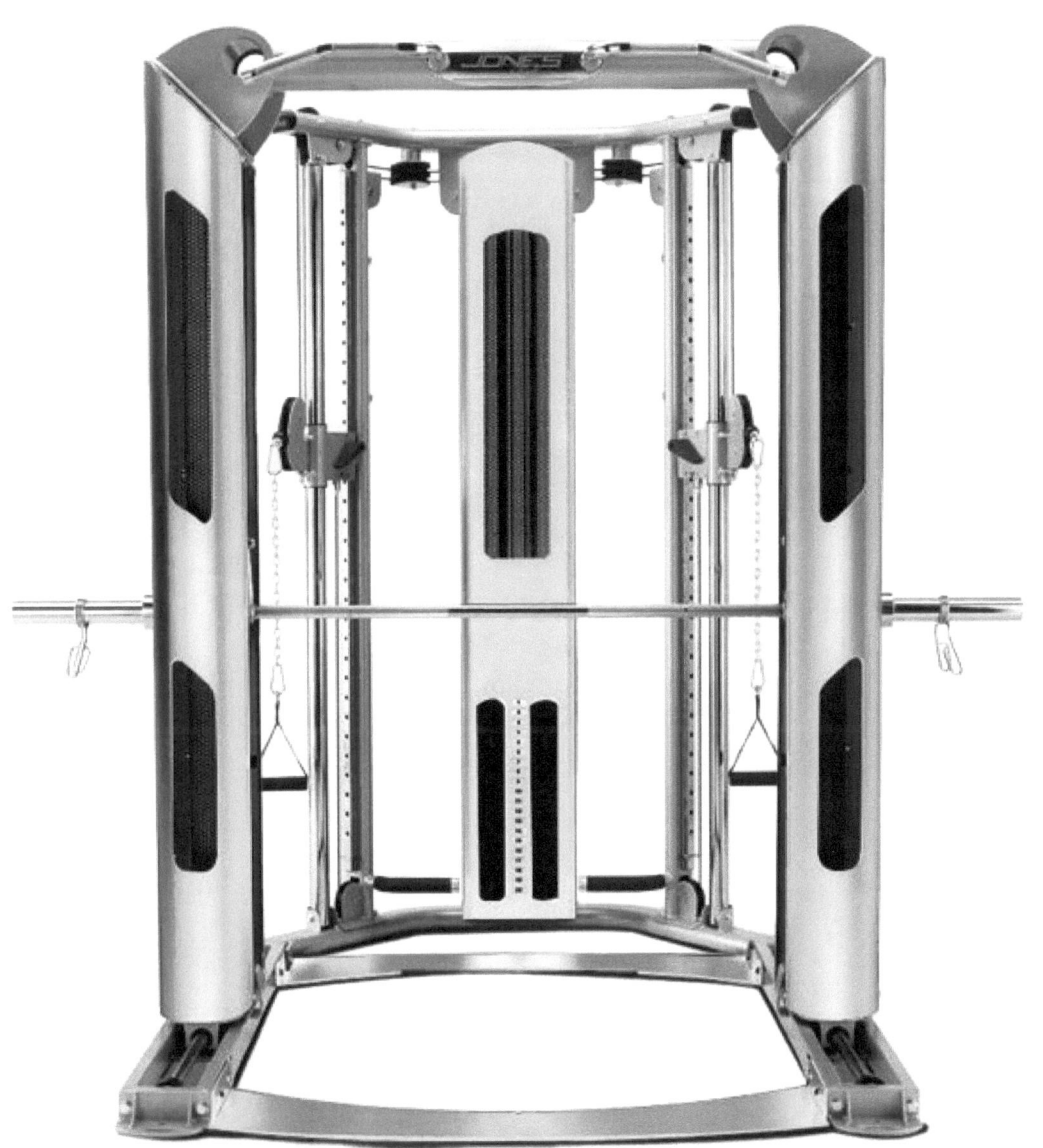

BODYCRAFT Jones Platinum

Chapter 3
Cardio Machines

No exercise routine would be complete without cardio. Cardio refers cardiovascular exercise and is essential to staying healthy and keeping fit. Many people, namely those looking to "bulk up," incorrectly believe that cardio will hinder their efforts at building muscle. However, cardio has multiple benefits, both for building muscle, "toning," staying healthy and building immunity to disease and illness.

Cardiovascular fitness can be defined as the strength of the heart muscles and its ability to provide oxygen to the rest of the body. Cardio improves heart health, endurance, and drastically reduces the likelihood of heart-related problems such as high blood pressure and high cholesterol. Cardio workouts also burn fat and increase the metabolism, helping build new muscle at a quicker pace. Cardio helps reduce fat mass built up from high-calorie diets needed for gaining hard muscle. Overall, cardio provides an increase in endurance and strength of the body and is essential

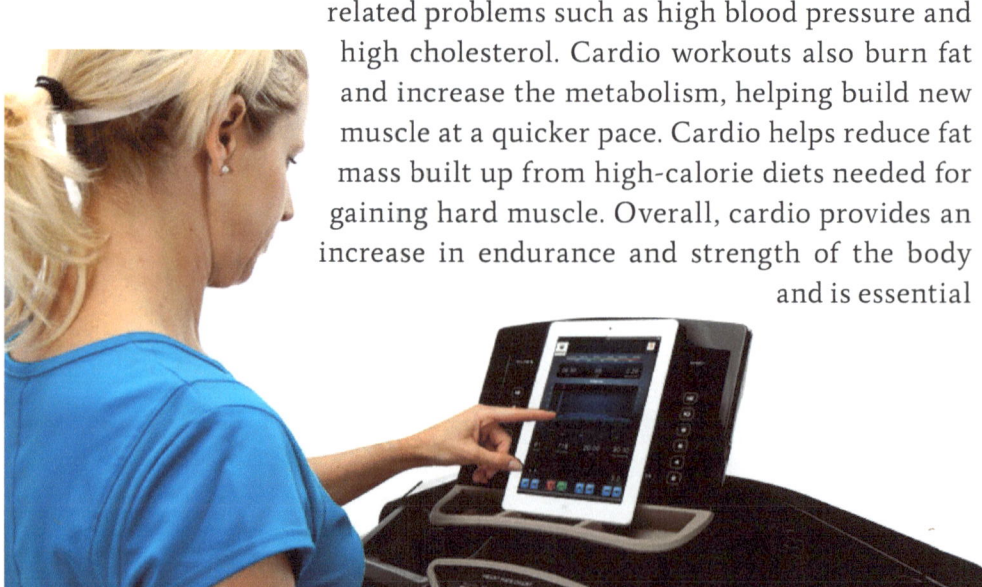

to any exercise routine. Therefore, incorporating cardio machines into your home gym is highly recommended.

But what machines should you get? How many machines? The world of cardio machines is a wide and confusing one to navigate. We've all seen the lone treadmill or stair climber gathering dust in someone's spare bedroom or garage. Obviously, you don't want your equipment to end up that way. That's why it's important to choose the cardio machine or machines that are right for your workout needs, your space restrictions, and your budget. But above all, the best cardio machine you can purchase is the one you're most willing to put to regular use.

Treadmills

The most stereotypical of exercise machines, treadmills have been symbolic of exercise and home gyms for decades. In fact, they're the single most used piece of exercise equipment. More than 50 million Americans use them, up nearly 40 percent in the last ten years. Treadmills burn the most calories of any of the cardiovascular machines. Walking briskly, you can expect to burn about 100 calories per mile, on average. But because treadmills are so common and there are literally thousands of options, and because they can be can be quite costly, it's important for you to consider carefully and choose the best one for your personal needs. So what do you look for in a treadmill? Consider the following criteria –

Your Goals: Before you begin your search, it's essential that you assess your goals and home situation. Are you the only individual that will be using the equipment? Or is it going to be a family item? Under buying, or buying an underpowered treadmill that will be used by a 140 pound person as well as a 240 pound person, is a common and avoidable mistake. Consider your own weight as one factor, but the more people and the more weight that will be placed on the machine, the more powerful and durable it will need to be.

Size: Treadmills can be both stationary and folding. Most treadmills are about 6.5 feet by 3 feet. Folding treadmills generally fold to about half their length but can still be quite large. Don't assume that you can simply tuck away a folding treadmill. A large treadmill, even folded, will still be bulky and might not fit into that closet you had in mind. Consider the size of the room you're planning to place the treadmill in. You need to be sure you have adequate space – roughly two feet on every side of the treadmill, to get on and off it safely.

Safety: You might not see treadmills as being a source of danger, but according to federal statistics, they're the single most dangerous piece of exercise equipment out there. In fact, injuries have gone up twofold in recent years. People have been known to break bones, scrape fingers, pull muscles and worse when working out on a treadmill. There are literally thousands of "funny" videos on Youtube showing people falling off treadmills and banging their heads against a wall or otherwise severely injuring themselves. Treadmill manufacturers have not been blind to the dangers associated with their equipment. Therefore, they long ago began incorporating safety features into their machines.

Practicality: Check your treadmills' deck length. Depending on what kind of exercise you want to do, you'll need a longer or shorter deck. A good treadmill should also offer adjustable strides. This is important if there will be more than one user. Also, when you walk, your gate is shorter than when you run. A stride adjustment will allow you to compensate for this.

Tech-features: Treadmills are more advanced than ever. You can find docks for tablets and music players, USB ports, TVs, and WiFi-enabled treadmills. Don't spend your money on these luxuries if you won't be using them. Buy the quality, durability and the features that you need and will use. Additional bells and whistles are a waste of your budget.

Assembly: Some treadmills can be extremely heavy, and many require assembly if you have them shipped directly to you. Some are more complicated than others but, generally, it takes a store technician 1 to 2 hours to put together a modern treadmill. If you're not particularly good with a toolbox, you might want to consider paying someone to accomplish this for you. Always ask about delivery and inquire whether assembly is included or available at additional cost.

Warranty: Most experts agree that purchasing an extended warranty is neither necessary nor generally worth the cost. Look for a treadmill that provides 2 to 5 years of warranty coverage on the motor and other main mechanics of the machine.

Your Needs: Consider what your fitness priorities are, and what your current fitness level is. Are you focused on losing weight, shredding, and/or building endurance? Then cardio should be the main focus of your workouts, in which case an investment in a top-tier treadmill is worth the extra expense. A good treadmill should last for years and you will find them priced between $1200 and $5000.

The main reason most people end up not using their treadmill is a lack of quality. We seem to have no qualms about investing in top-of-the-line golf clubs or outdoor bicycles, or paying for heated seats in our new cars. But when it comes to choosing fitness equipment, people want to spend the least possible amount. You need to avoid this kind of thinking or you will end up regretting your purchase. Remember that you should be using this piece of equipment three times a week for many years. If it doesn't provide you with a quiet, comfortable running experience, you will abandon it after a short time and it will become a wasted investment.

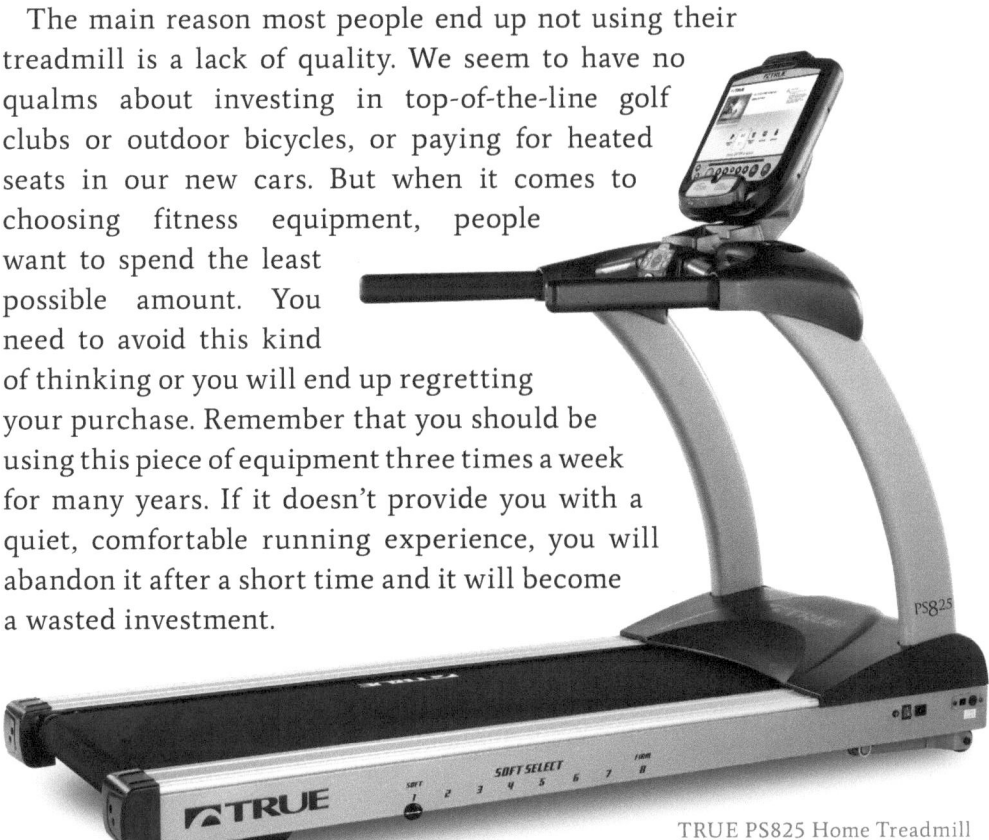

TRUE PS825 Home Treadmill

Ellipticals

The elliptical machine is gaining in use and popularity. While still trailing the treadmill, the elliptical is one of the most popular machines out there. Combining movements from stair climbing with cross country skiing, it's a great way to get a lower body workout along with your cardio, and they can be a bit more interesting than running or walking in a straight line. Some people prefer different motions for exercising their legs and it's good to switch things up! You might consider purchasing both a treadmill and an elliptical for your home gym. Many of the features that you want in a treadmill also apply to an elliptical, but here are some additional features to look for –

Smoothness: The purpose of an elliptical is to provide a simulation for running that doesn't involve as much impact. It's great for people with sensitive knees or fragile bones. When choosing an elliptical, get a feel for the machine. We mean that literally. The elliptical motion should be completely smooth. When the heel comes off the platform, you shouldn't feel any kicks or bounces. When moving, you should be able to exercise in a neutral position without having to grasp for the handrails or reach over.

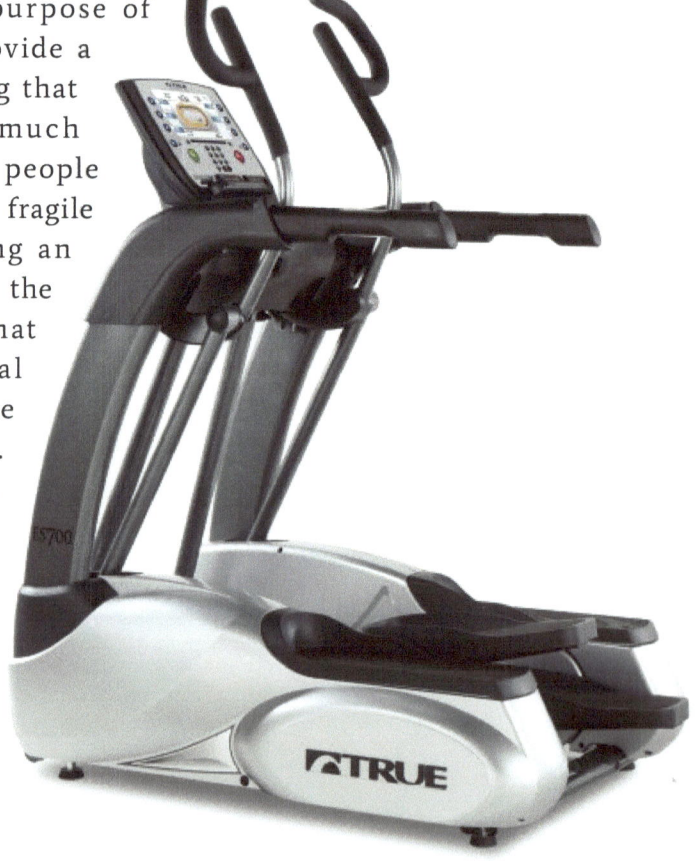

TRUE ES700 Home Elliptical Trainer

Range of Motion: Your elliptical should be able to move both forwards and backwards. Forward and reverse motions allow you to add variety to your workout and challenge yourself.

Resistance: Resistance levels should be adjustable. You want your elliptical to grow with you. As your legs become more powerful, you'll need to increase the resistance on the machine. If your workout is no longer challenging, it is no longer effective.

Tech-features: As with a treadmill, consider the benefit of tech features such as iPad - iPhone docking stations, TVs, and Wi-Fi capability. Being able to watch a television show or listen to music while working out helps pass by the time and can even make your workout fun! But, as mentioned earlier, bells and whistles that you will not use are an unnecessary drain on your budget that would be better spent on other equipment or accessories.

Manufacturers are innovating all the time, seeking to improve performance, effectiveness and comfort for the user. TRUE fitness, a higher-end equipment maker now offers their patented Core Drive™ system. Rather than a front drive or rear drive system, Core drive places the drive directly beneath your feet. This, according to TRUE, means you no longer have to put pressure on the front of your toes which, in turn, puts pressure on the knees. TRUE maintains that this provides the most natural movement and keeps the user in the center of the exercise motion for superior balance, stability and comfort. If this interests you, find a facility where you can test this claim for yourself to see if it provides an improved workout experience.

Cost: The more features the elliptical has, the more it will cost. Still, even the best ellipticals won't top $8000. Many people love their ellipticals and do most or all of their cardio workouts on it. If you like the motion of an elliptical, or have sensitive joints, a higher tier elliptical is probably for you. Fun features like iPod docks and even cooling fans will give you a nice return on your investment entertainment-wise, as they'll help the time fly by!

Exercise Bikes

With the advent of spin classes and music-inspired workouts, exercise bikes have soared in popularity. Exercise bikes look deceptively simple but, when done right, there is no other machine that will get you sweating as much as this one! But, of course, with the explosion in popularity also came an explosion in additional features. It can be hard to distinguish between all the different bikes. Here's a breakdown. There are five basic types of exercise bike: upright stationary bikes, recumbent stationary bikes, dual-action stationary bikes, indoor cycles, and interactive stationary bikes. When picking a bike, look for ones that feel smooth and comfortable to you. Remember, you'll be sitting on your bike for long periods of time so you want to be sure it's comfortable!

BODYCRAFT SPT
Indoor Club Group Cycle

Upright Exercise Bikes: These are most like traditional bicycles and the simplest of exercise bikes. They have seats and pedals just like normal bicycles and the feel of riding them is the same as riding a real bicycle. Sometimes they'll include added features like distance tracking and adjustable resistance. They are usually the smallest of bikes and so are easy to store. They are also relatively inexpensive compared to some of the other types.

Recumbent Stationary Bikes: These bikes are similar to normal upright bikes, but have wider seats and backrests. The rider is slightly reclined, with the bike pedals in front of the seat instead of below the seat. Recumbent bikes are popular among people who prefer additional back support and comfort. Picture lifting your legs in front of you and pedaling. This will utilize more muscle groups, including the abdominals and glutes, for a more complete workout. They're also a great option if you're one of those people who likes to read while cycling.

Dual-action Stationary Bikes: These are for people seeking a full-body workout. Dual-action bikes work out both the upper and lower bodies. Like ellipticals, dual-action bikes have handlebars that move in sync with the pedals. This constant motion of the arms increases aerobic intensity, provides additional exercise, and gets your blood flowing all-around.

Indoor Cycles: These guys are what you'd typically see in a spin class room. These are similar to upright exercise bikes but are much sleeker and simpler. The resistance of the pedals can be adjusted, but other than that, indoor cycles are mostly bare-bones. That is, they

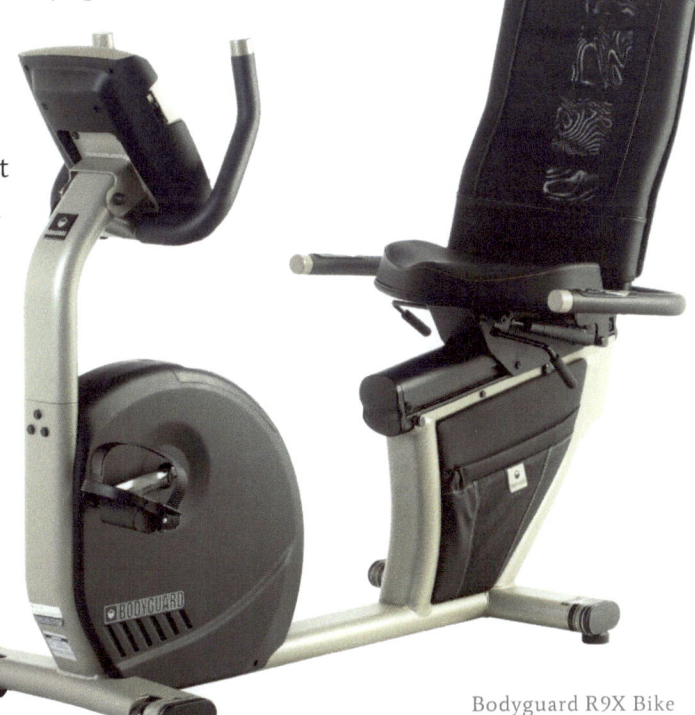

Bodyguard R9X Bike

don't usually include features such as calorie or distance trackers. However, indoor cycles provide the most intense workout.

Interactive Stationary Bikes: These are the most high-tech of the bunch, allowing riders to combine the wonders of technology with their workout. These bikes can have anything from computers to televisions. Some even feature computer-generated fitness programs that structure workouts and make them more entertaining. Often, you'll have an array of options to choose from, such as endurance training, weight loss, interval training, and more.

How do you decide how much money to put into a bike? Consider just how often you'll use it. As seen with the popularity of spin classes, some people love their spinners. They can easily turn into a fun and healthy fitness addiction. If you're looking for a one-piece cardio "wow" item, go for a quality bike.

Rowing Machines

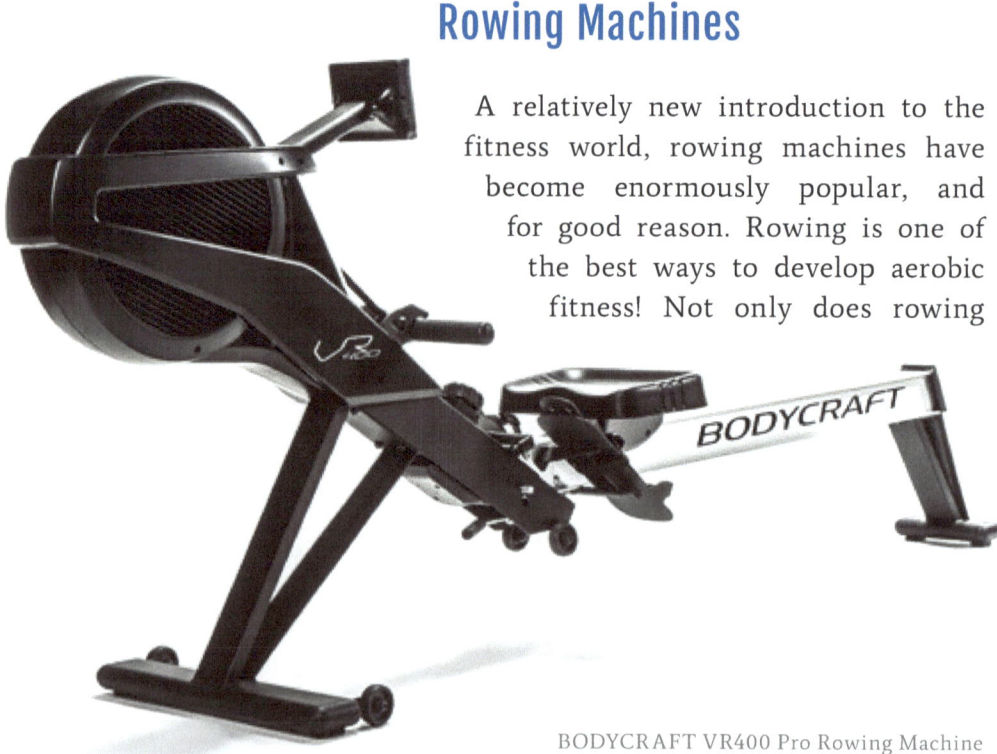

A relatively new introduction to the fitness world, rowing machines have become enormously popular, and for good reason. Rowing is one of the best ways to develop aerobic fitness! Not only does rowing

BODYCRAFT VR400 Pro Rowing Machine

provide great cardio, but it strengthens the muscles of your upper and lower body as well. With a rowing machine, you can quickly burn fat while getting toned arms, legs, shoulders and increasing core balance, all while adding fun variety to your workout. It's a great option for people who have sore or injured joints which can be uncomfortably jostled on treadmills or other cardio machines.

There are four types of indoor rowing machines: hydraulic rowing machines, flywheel rowing machines, magnetic resistance indoor rowing machines, and water rowing machines.

Hydraulic Rowing Machines: Hydraulic rowing machines provide resistance by air that is compressed with a cylinder or piston. This tension can be adjusted for added difficulty. Hydraulic rowing machines are ideal for people looking for a low-cost, space-saving solution. The one drawback to hydraulic rowers, however, is that the rowing machine technique doesn't allow you to pull a straight line – that is, it does not allow you to perform a natural rowing motion. Because of this, you'll get a less effective lower body workout than you would with actual rowing. In fact, with "real" rowing and with other rowing machines, your rowing workout is composed of approximately 65% to 75% legwork and 25% to 35% upper body work. With a hydraulic rowing machine, these percentages are reversed. Hydraulic rowing machines are the most economical of all rowing machines, and cost anywhere between $800 and $2000. They are ideal for the beginning rower.

Flywheel Rowing Machines: Flywheel rowers provide exercise that feels similar to outdoor rowing. It receives its resistance from the pulling motion which spins a flywheel. The flywheel provides resistance by moving against the wind it generates. To increase the resistance of a flywheel rower, you simply pull harder to move the flywheel faster. Flywheels provide a sweeping, smoother feel to rowing than hydraulic rowers. Flywheels are good for fitness enthusiasts, or people who are relatively experienced at rowing. A good quality flywheel rower will cost between $500 and $1500.

Magnetic Resistance Indoor Rowing Machines: Magnetic resistance rowers are popular because they are virtually silent and are extremely smooth. As their name implies, magnetic resistance rowers use a magnetic brake system to develop resistance. Magnetic resistance rowers are a common purchase, and can be used by amateurs and experts alike. They cost between $600 and $1800.

Water Rowing Machine: The water rower is most similar to outdoor rowing, and ideal for rowers who wish to train for their sport and practice in the off-season. The water rower is designed to simulate the dynamics of a boat moving through water, and like the magnetic rower, is essentially soundless. Most water rowers have a wooden frame, to resemble boats. They are the most expensive of the rowing machines, costing $1000 and up, and also take up the most space. But for a dedicated rower or fitness enthusiast, a water rower is a powerful and fun way to work out.

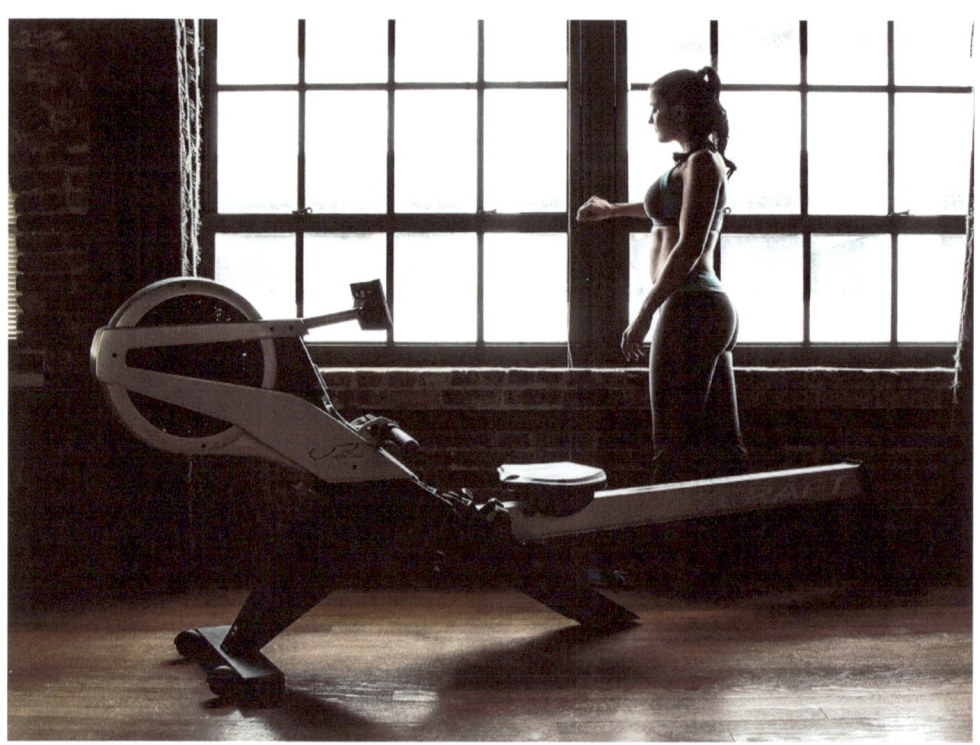

BODYCRAFT VR500 Pro Rowing Machine

Chapter 4
Free Weights: Dumbbells, Barbells, Kettlebells, etc.

If you think you don't need free weights in your gym, you are incorrect. Strength training is an absolute must for any exercise routine, and nothing is better than free weights when it comes to strength training. Strength training is for both men and women, regardless of their fitness goals. It'll get you stronger, leaner, and healthier.

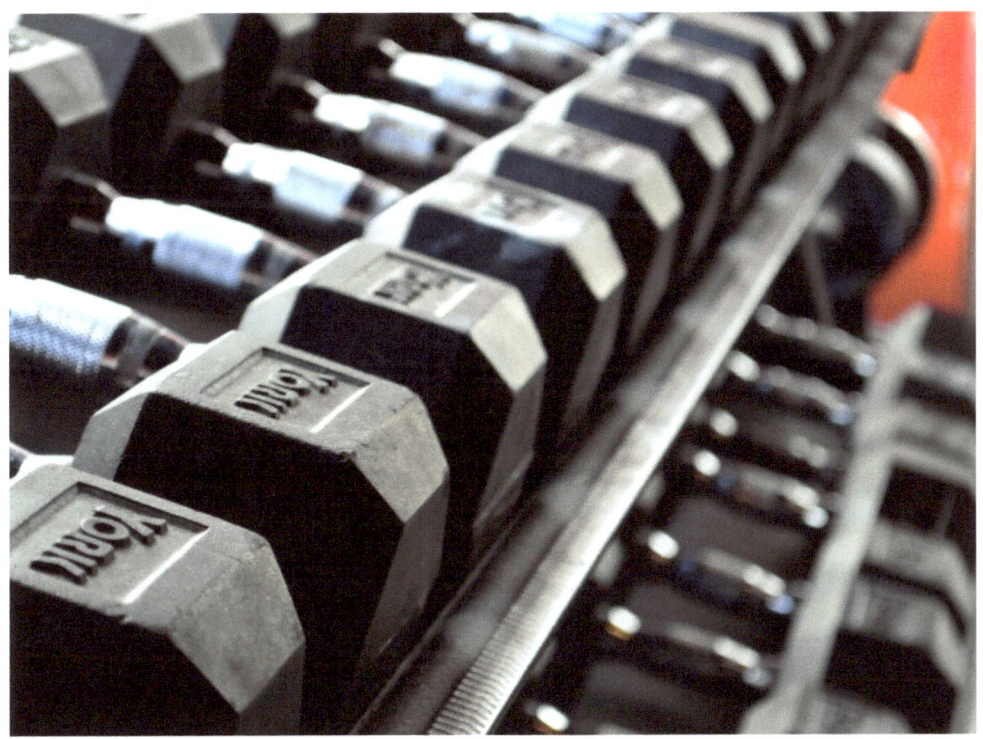

Photo by Aberro Creative

Here are some of the benefits of strength training:

- **Developing Stronger Bones:** By actually putting your bones to work, free-weight training increases your bone density and reduces the risk of osteoporosis and injury.

- **Lose Weight:** The more muscle you gain, the less fat you have. And the more muscle you have, the more your body begins to burn calories more efficiently, pulling from those fat stores everybody wants to get rid of.

- **Boost Stamina and Endurance:** Building muscle contributes to better balance and more power. As you get stronger, you will fatigue less easily. This is especially beneficial as investment against the strain of time. You'll be much fitter and mobile in old age if you strength train!

- **Become Healthier:** Strength training with free weights can reduce symptoms of many chronic conditions such as back pain, arthritis, and heart disease.

So how do you build up the perfect collection of free-weights? First know that there are different types of free weights. Dumbbells and barbells are the classic strength training tools, but there are also kettlebells.

Dumbbells

These are probably the most versatile of free weights and the best choice for a beginner. Dumbbells are about 10 to 15 inches long and are held in one hand. They can be either fixed-weight or adjustable. Adjustable are short, straight bars with weight plates, usually in 5 pound increments. Adjustable dumbbells tend to be cheaper but they are also clunkier and can be less comfortable to use. They tend to be made out of metal, with metal grips. If you're keeping your weights outside, these might not be your best option, as they tend to rust.

Fixed-weight Dumbbells: Fixed-weight dumbbells can come in multiple shapes and materials. The most common materials are rubber and chrome. They also come with ends in two primary shapes: hexagonal and circular.

Between the two shapes there is only one primary difference besides aesthetics: practicality.

Hexagonal shaped dumbbells are less likely to roll away when you set them on the floor, which can save you the pain of accidentally tripping over one or having one roll over your toes! In terms of materials, it's really a matter of personal preference. Test both metal and neoprene and see which grip you like more.

Neoprene is generally easier to hold, but is uncomfortable for some. However, neoprene is much more practical for outdoor gyms, as neoprene dumbbells won't rust. If you're getting fixed-weight dumbbells, be sure to buy a few different sets of weights. You will quickly outgrow one weight set, so get 2 or 3 sets of dumbbells above your current preferred weight. For example, if you're currently training with 10 pound dumbbells, consider buying 15 pound, 20 pound and 25 pound sets as well. This will be a little more costly, but also more practical in that it will ensure that you don't outgrow the effectiveness of your dumbbell workout quickly.

Single sets of dumbbells start at approximately $15 and go up as the weight goes up. On average, expect to pay at least $45 for a set of dumbbells over 15 pounds. If you want a complete dumbbell kit—that is, with multiple sets — that are all above 15 pounds, you'll need to put down $700 to $1000 and up. The good news is that you likely don't need weights over 50 pounds unless you're already an accomplished lifter.

Adjustable Dumbbells: If you don't mind "fiddling" around with weights a bit and you want to save some money, consider a set of adjustable dumbbells. Some consider them less comfortable to work with but they will still get the job done and a single set of adjustable dumbbells will grow with you. If you don't plan to use weights too often, or only wish to use them for a handful of exercises which you want to get better at, go for adjustable dumbbells. You can get a decent set (up to 50 pounds usually) for $350. These are a good option if you don't have a lot of money to spend, don't have a lot of space, or want to test the waters before diving all the way in.

Barbells

Barbells are long metal bars with weights at each end. They are lifted with both hands for equal weight distribution across the spine. Barbells are a great way to add variety to your workout and they have as many unique exercises as dumbbells. There's a reason why barbells are so popular with bodybuilders – they are the tools of the big boys and they really work. But because barbells are the heavy-hitters, they can also be more dangerous. Don't invest in barbells until you're ready for them and don't try to lift them before you are instructed in proper usage. Using barbells incorrectly can easily lead to muscle injury or, worse, a banged up head or foot as a result of a barbell falling on you. When you're ready for barbells, here's what you'll need –

Bars: These hold the barbell together and they are between 4 and 7 feet long. They come in two sizes: standard (25 pounds) and olympic (45 pounds). Olympic bars are the bars most commonly found in gyms, mostly because they are easier to hold and more comfortable. Most standard barbells can hold up to 200 pounds but Olympic barbells can handle loads over 800 pounds. Bars come with threaded or unthreaded ends. With threaded ends, the plates are held in place with spinlocks that are screwed on. With unthreaded, the plates are squeezed or slipped on. There are two key things to avoid when shopping for bars; hollow bars and bars that must be assembled from pieces. Neither is sturdy enough to hold heavy weights and if the bar buckles, you'll be in danger.

Plates and Collars: Plates are the round weights that you slide onto the bars and collars are the clips used to secure the plates in place. Both plates and collars are designed to specifically fit either a standard bar or an olympic bar, so be sure that you buy plates and collars that match the size of your bar. A good strategy is to buy a bar that comes with a number of weight plates included. This will provide you with a "starter set" that should suffice until you're more comfortable with barbells and are ready to move up with more weight.

Racks: You'll need a rack to store your plates and bars. A good choice is to buy a power rack with sections on which you can set your barbell above your head. This will allow you to use your barbell set without the help of a spotter. There are also a variety of racks for storing barbells, weight plates, dumbbells, etc. when they are not in use. A rack is about $70 and up – more expensive for more tiers.

Sets: You can also buy barbells that already come with all the necessary components. This is the best option for beginners or those simply looking for simplicity. You can get a 50 to 100 pound barbell set for as little as $175. Even barbell sets up to a few hundred pounds shouldn't run you much more than $600.

Benches: Lastly, but essentially, you'll need a bench. Weight benches come in all shapes and sizes. Make sure your bench is wide enough to

Jordan Studio Barbell Rack

support you, that it doesn't wobble, and that it's sturdy enough to hold you and the weight you're trying to lift. Avoid collapsible benches if possible. While they may seem ideal for saving space, they're only recommended if you plan to lift a minimal amount of weight. A nice investment is an adjustable incline bench. This will allow you to do strength training focused on your shoulders and upper pectorals. Other types of benches include those with leg extension and curl features. Some of these actually bend, allowing you to get in a leg workout, while some only offer a better grip. You may find these type of benches more or less comfortable than a simpler one. If you're looking to knock out two birds with one stone, you can also find a weight bench that comes with an adjustable rack.

If you don't plan to lift weights heavier than 50 pounds, or you're not really a serious lifter, a standard bench should suit you just find. You can get a decent bench for around $350 — no need to shell out a lot of money for this one. If you're planning to bulk up via weightlifting, you'll need something sturdier under your back. A bargain weight bench may turn out to be dangerous if you're straining it with a lot weight. Go for a bench that's between $250 and $750. These will be heavy enough to withstand more weight and will have adjustable neck and back support too. Whatever you choose, always shop with an eye to quality and safety over price considerations alone.

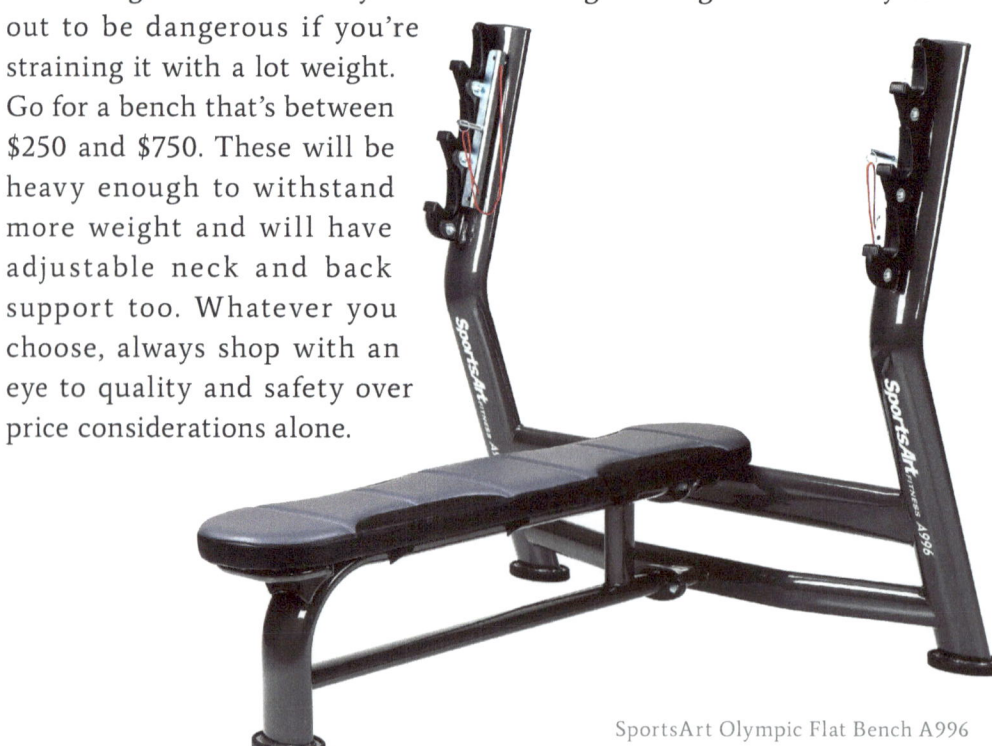

SportsArt Olympic Flat Bench A996

Kettlebells

Kettlebells have recently come into fashion, but they've quickly risen to the top of the list of most effective exercise routines. They can be used for ballistic lifts, such as swings, cleans, snatches, tossing, and juggling, or grinds such as overhead presses, dead-lifts, windmills, and more. Kettlebells make for an excellent and effective workout.

Things to look for when shopping for kettlebells – weight, grip, shape, and material. First of all, be conservative in the initial weight you choose. It's easy to think you are stronger than you are and pick a kettlebell that is too heavy for you. Exercising with an oversized kettlebell is dangerous and you can end up with a pulled muscle or worse. Pick a reasonable size. For ballistic movements, average men should start out with a 35 or 45 pound kettlebell. More athletic men can start anywhere between a 35 pound and 62 pound kettlebell. For grinding movements, choose a kettlebell you can easily press overhead about 10 times. This would be between 18 and 26 pounds for the average man and between 26 and 44 pounds for an active one.

Average women pursuing ballistic movements should aim for a kettlebell between 18 and 26 pounds. An athletic woman should start with a kettlebell between 26 and 35 pounds. For grinding movements, an average woman should begin with a kettlebell between 13 and 18 pounds, while an athletic one should work with one between 18 and 26 pounds.

Pick a kettlebell that you can get a good grip on, one whose shape fits against your forearm well, and a material that is both aesthetically pleasing and practical for you. A metal kettlebell might not be as comfortable and it might easily rust outdoors. On the other hand, a metal kettlebell is less prone than a rubber one to scratches and dirt. If you want to really "tone" your muscles and you don't plan to invest in exercise machines, a kettlebell will be a great addition to your workout. A kettlebell can be less than $20 to over $100 depending on its weight. It will fill in the gaps when it comes to muscles you might otherwise miss with free weights. Kettlebells are great for exercisers of any proficiency. Poke around and read reviews to find the best type and brand for your intended use.

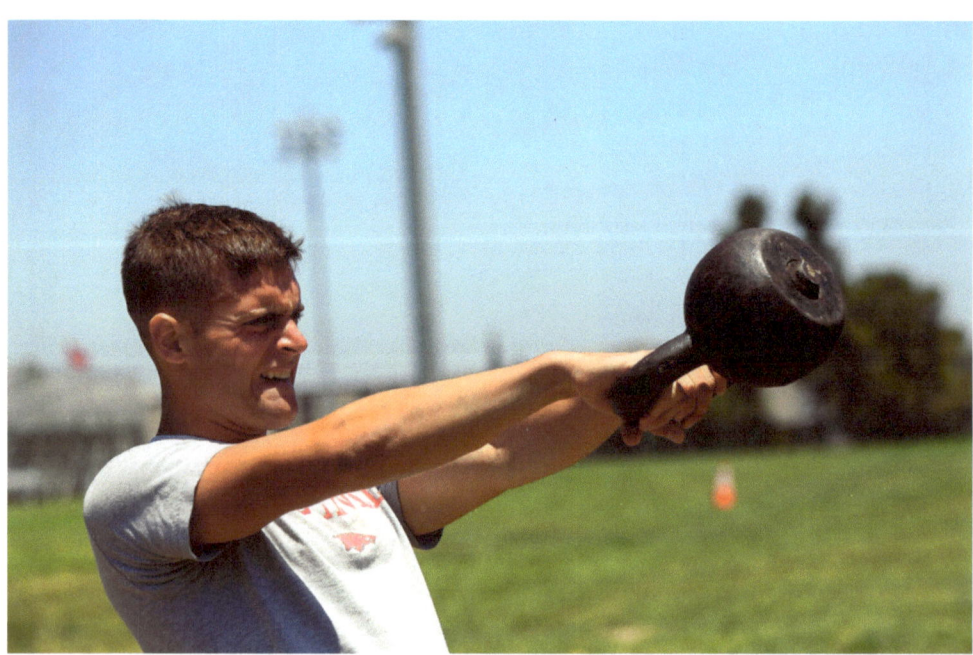

Lance Cpl. Ben Lowry, assistant gunner with Low Altitude Air Defence Battalion, Marine Air Wing, performs kettle-bell exercises during the Cobat Conditioning Training Course at the Paige Field House on Marine Corps Base Camp Pendleton, July 24.
Photo by: Lance Cpl. Sarah Wolff-Diaz

Chapter 5
Chin Up and Pull Up Bars

Though they may look easy, chin ups and pull ups are actually difficult to do. And while they are difficult, they're some of the best exercises out there and can get your arms and shoulders really burning. Consistent exercise with chin up and pull up bars will leave you with cut arms and shoulders and powerful upper body strength. Whether or not you're currently at the level where you're able to do chin ups and pull ups, a chin up or pull up bar is an excellent investment. Relatively inexpensive and easy to install, these bars offer a multitude of exercise options and a great way to track your progress (one week you can do only 5 pull-ups and three months later you can do 25 – progress achieved). In fact, bars are one of the cheapest and best ways to build strength and definition in your back, arms and shoulders! There are several types of doorway bars and a few things to look for.

Doorway Bars: You've seen doorway pull up bars everywhere from movies to the bedrooms of teenage boys. You might have also seen videos of unfortunate souls breaking their doors or falling to the floor when their doorway bar buckles. Doorway bars may not be as ideal as a full-fledged pull up machine, but they're not quite as fickle as media makes them out to be either.

Over the Door Pull Up Bars: These go over the top of the doorframe and leverage your weight to stay in place. You hook the frame to your door and once you're finished with your workout, you can unhook the bar and stow it out of sight. Leverage bars typically come in pieces which are easy to assemble, typically with a provided throw-away wrench. Assembly should take about 10 to 15 minutes. Over the door bars are probably the most sturdy, though also more expensive. They generally have a weight limit of around 300 pounds and range in price from around $40 to $100.

Mounted Pull Up Bars: If you're lucky enough to have a space specifically designated for your home gym, or you don't mind a more permanent bar, consider a mounted pull up bar. These bars mount directly to a brick wall or to the studs behind drywall. They can be mounted to either wall or ceiling. These are a bit more expensive, but generally more reliable. They do require more installation time, however, and you should be careful to align them parallel to the ground. A crooked bar is going to give you a crooked workout and possibly result in muscle injury. If you're serious about fitness and building your own home gym (and don't mind drilling into your wall), go for a mounted pull up bar. Even if you can't use it right away, you'll find that it will soon become one of your most-used items as you get stronger! There's almost no better exercise to build up arm strength and muscle than a pull up. These can go for as much as $300.

Free Standing Pull Up Bars: Free standing pull up bars can be several feet tall and are quite heavy. They work by being big and heavy enough to support your weight. These are the most expensive option, $600 or more, but they also have the advantage of having multiple fixtures, such as arm rests, which allow you to do many additional exercises. Arm rests are particularly advantageous for core exercises such as leg raises. Free standing pull up bars are an ideal choice for anyone who has the money. You can do a lot of different exercises on them — both beginners AND experts — and the added diversity to your workout will make it well worth your money.

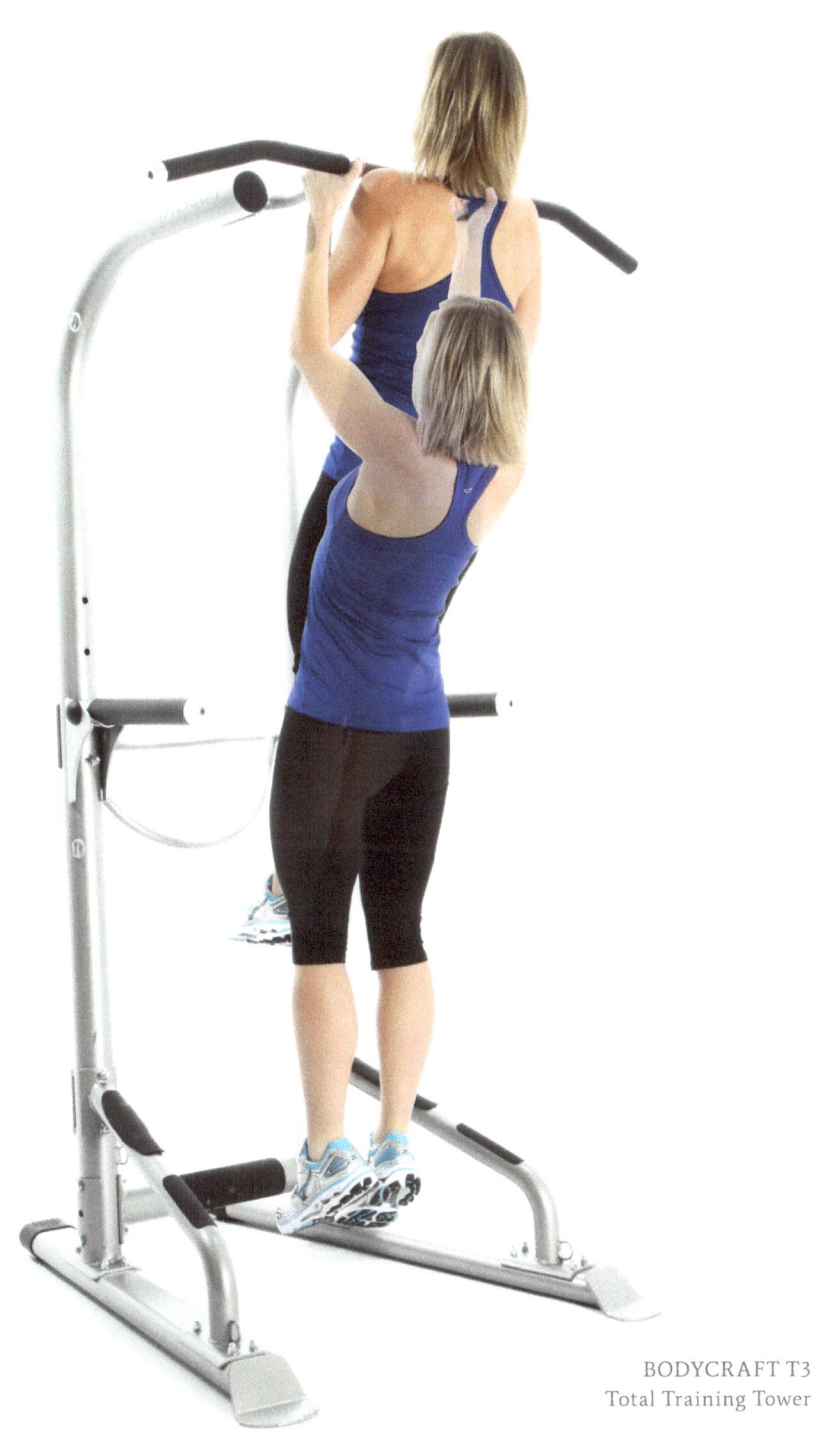

BODYCRAFT T3
Total Training Tower

Chapter 6
Workout Machines: Legs and Lower Body

Now, on to the big boys — the workout machines. While you can easily create a great workout routine with no machines at all, most people find machines help them to add variety and simplicity to their workout. When it comes to leg machines, there are dozens of options and you might find it confusing trying to decide which are going to give you the best results, and which are most worth their purchase price. We've outlined the most common types of leg machines and their benefits relative to cost.

Leg Press Machines: One of the best workout machines for an overall lower body workout is the leg press. Not only does

SportsArt Leg Press A982

it tone and firm up your legs, it works out all of your lower body muscles as well. It's especially good for your butt. It's also one of the safer machines to use, as weight cannot fall back down on you. Leg presses, however, can be extremely heavy and can run up to the thousands of dollars, depending on how intricate the machine is. If you're just starting out, a simple machine, which should cost less than $2000, is all you'll need. If you're looking for more complicated movements and higher weight levels, consider investing in a more sophisticated and heavy-duty machine. A leg press machine, while nice, isn't necessary for the beginner. For those just doing moderate exercise, you can work out your legs in many other ways. Leg presses are good for bodybuilders and gym rats who want to really beef up their legs by weightlifting.

Leg Curl/Extension Machines: Leg curl machines exercise hamstrings and leg extension machines help develop shapely thighs while strengthening the knees. Unless you intend to curl/extend very high weight levels, your best bet is to choose a two-in-one machine, which offers both the leg curl and the leg extension options. Most machines found at commercial gyms are combination curl and extension machines. A combo machine is the best bet for the average person, and it's one

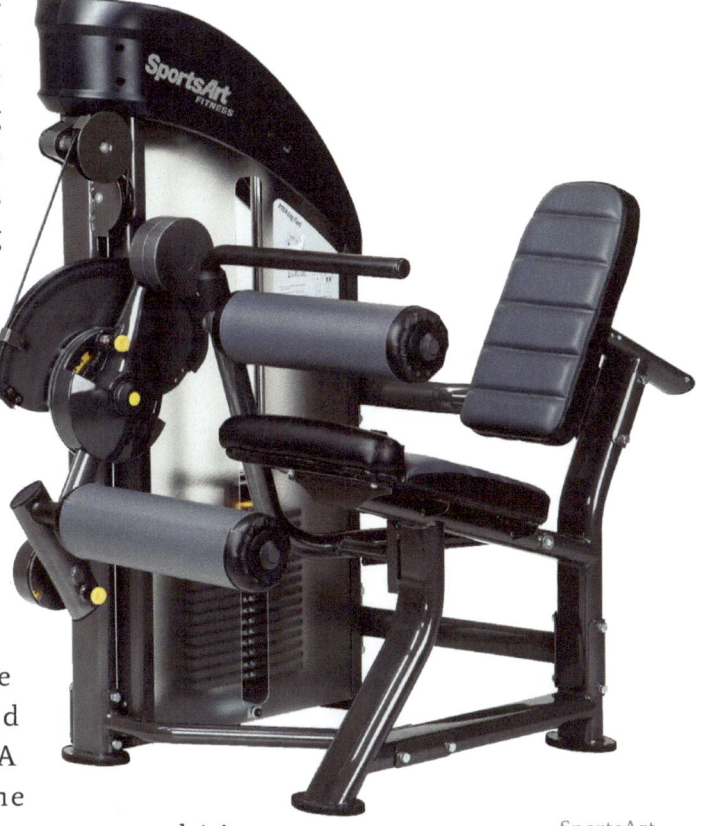

SportsArt
Leg Curl P759

of the most useful leg exercise machines out there. In fact, if you're only going to get one leg machine, get this. You'll get a gut-busting workout of your quadriceps, glutes, hamstrings, calves, and abductors (i.e. most muscles from your calves to your waist). It's a guarantee you'll be feeling this one in the morning!

Calf Bench: With this machine, you use your calf muscles to push the resistance pads outwards. This one is easy to use but hard to master, and will really get your calf muscles burning. No matter what level of fit you're at, the calf bench will help you strengthen your lower legs. The cheapest calf benches run about $350. More intricate ones with higher weight levels go for $300 to $2000.

You really don't need more machines than this to get a burning workout and really put your lower body to the test. Other exercises

SportsArt Seated Calf Raise A981

beneficial to leg toning and strengthening either use free weight exercises, such as calf raises, or body resistance exercises like lunges and squats.

Chapter 7
Workout Machines: Upper Body and Abs

Everyone wants rocking abs and burgeoning biceps. Even if you're only looking to cut and define, upper body and ab machines will help you get toned and fit. Upper body machines are sturdy investments. Here are some of the best machines out there for targeting your chest, biceps, triceps, abs, back, and shoulders.

Horizontal Chest Press: This machine simulates a bench press, working out the chest, triceps and shoulders. This is a great way to get a chest workout if you don't have a set of barbells or don't want to use barbells without a spotter. You should only buy a chest press if you're really serious about fitness and want to put your money behind that belief. Chest press machines start at a minimum of $450 and go up to $3000. Only buy it if you plan to get full use out of this machine. If you plan to really bulk up, invest in a solid machine with a high range of weights. This will be more expensive, but will provide you with a good workout all throughout your fitness journey.

SportsArt Dependent Chest Press P715

Seated High Row: High row machines workout the back and biceps simultaneously, which helps strengthen upper body balance. High rows can strengthen hard-to-reach lower lat muscles and are ideal for beginners to weight training who want to develop a strong back. It will strengthen the back and prepare you for more advanced weight exercises. Beginners need an inexpensive machine with a relatively small range of weights. Such machines are $1000 and up. More advanced users might want a great set of weights, in which case they might spend $3000 and up for a good machine.

Lat Pull Down: The lat pull down is a popular machine, even for bodybuilders who prefer free weights, and for good reason. This one consists of a machine with a seat and a wide bar attached to the top pulley. Essentially a reverse pull up, a lat pull down increases the width and definition of the back. It's particularly effective for the lower back, and it also works out core muscles, which help balance you as you pull down on the bar. Most lat machines will offer different grips to target different muscles. A lat pull down machine is a great choice for anyone, regardless of level of fitness. Between $1200 to $4000, they are a bit of an investment, but you'll be using this all throughout your fitness regime.

Seated Shoulder Press: This machine is excellent for working out your shoulder muscles and your triceps. It is a common machine in gyms and

SportsArt Lat Pull Down S926

exercise clubs, and for good reason. It mimics a free weight shoulder press to strengthen the deltoid muscle. It widens your back and makes it feel and look stronger. Regular exercise with this machine also helps eliminate lower back pain, which some people experience when doing shoulder presses with free weights. This machine will cost you at least $400. It can be used by anyone, regardless of fitness level. If you suffer from lower back pain, this might be a beneficial machine for you to have. Bodybuilders might prefer free weights for building their shoulder muscles and triceps.

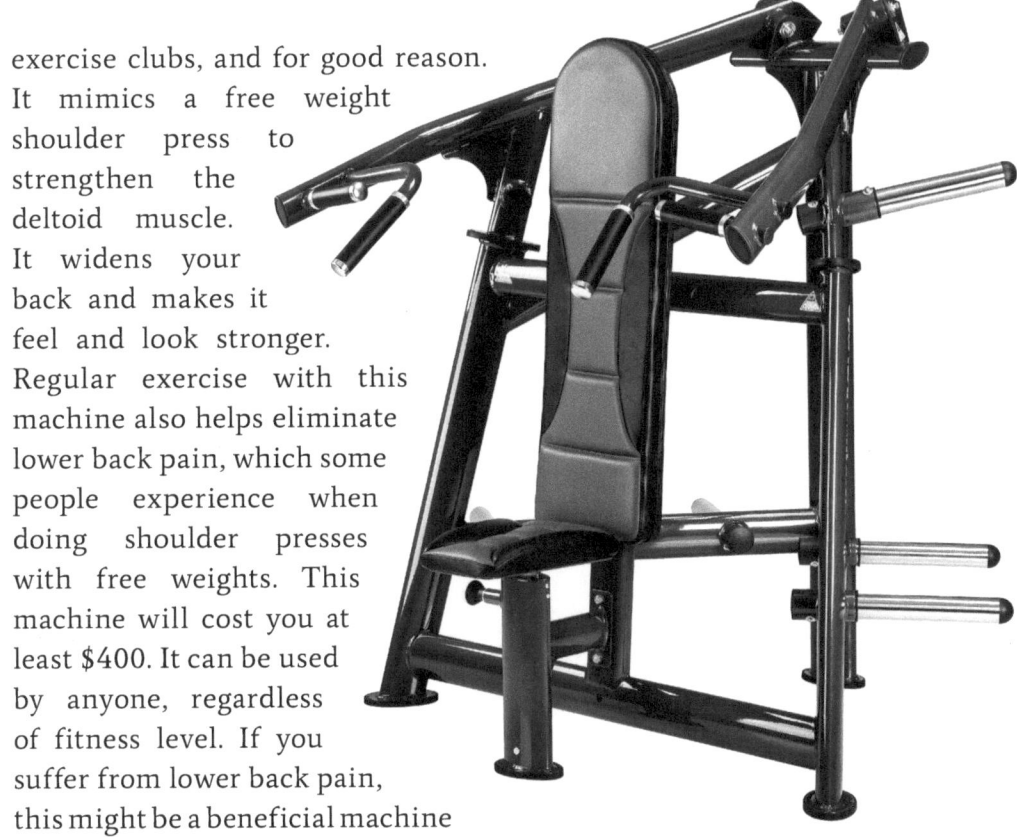

SportsArt Shoulder Press A987

Pec Fly: These imitate dumbbell chest flys and target the pectoral muscles in the chest. They also work out the deltoid muscle and the serrates muscles in the ribcage. The pec fly machine is a great choice for anyone looking to toughen up those hard-to-target pec muscles and to expand their chest. Pectoral muscles are some of the most noticeable parts of the upper body, so by really working out this set of muscles, you can positively influence your physique. Stereotypes aside, men usually prefer this machine as it adds some solidity to their pecs, making for a good upper body look. A pec fly machine will run you at least $3000. But for beginner and bodybuilder alike, this is a solid use of funds!

Tricep Dip: This is a small bar set on which you push off with your arms. It targets your tricep muscles, those sometimes pesky muscles on the back of your upper arms. A tricep dip machine is a good investment for anyone at any level of fitness, but you might not need one if you buy a free-standing pull up machine which includes tricep dip bars. A free-standing pull up machine is considerably more expensive, however, while a tricep dip bar set will only run you between $100 and $200.

Bicep Curl Machine: If you prefer machines to free weights, the bicep curl machine is a must. Bicep curl machines isolate the biceps and help build bulging muscles. These machines are ideal for both beginners and expert body lifters. Beginners have the benefit of having trained and safe movement (it's easy to incorrectly use free weights), while experts get the framework support of the machine, which allows them to lift higher amounts of weight. These machines are an investment,

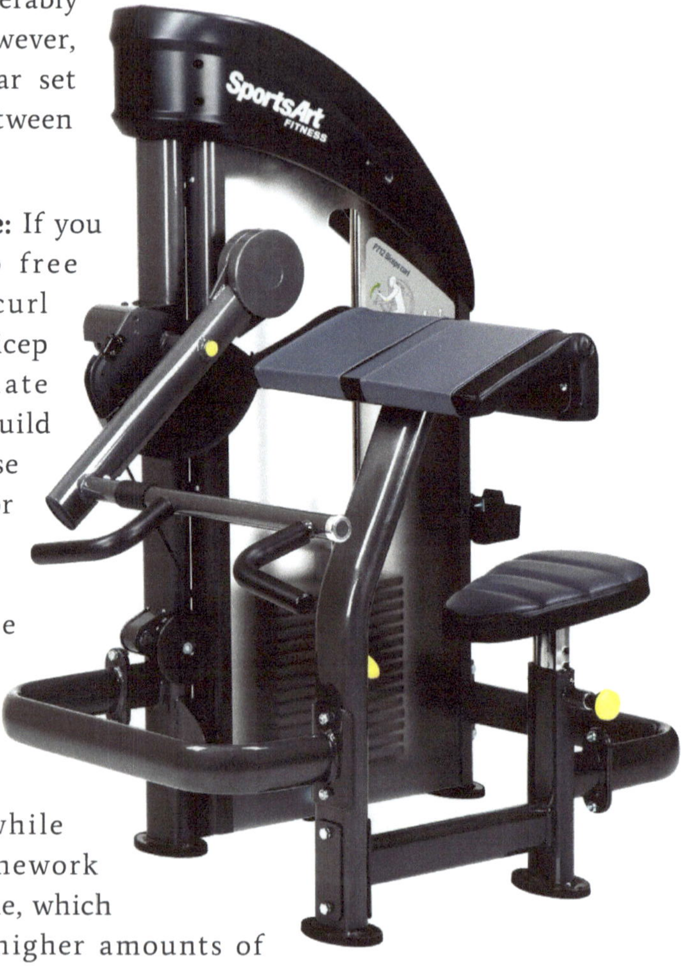

SportsArt Biceps Curl P712

42

though, and the cheapest of them start at about $300. They can easily run up to $3000.

Abdominal Crunch Machine: This is where your 6 pack or more defined abs start. A crunch machine is easy, effective, and safer than free weight exercises. This is because a crunch machine avoids tweaking your neck at strange angles, keeping you from feeling sore later.

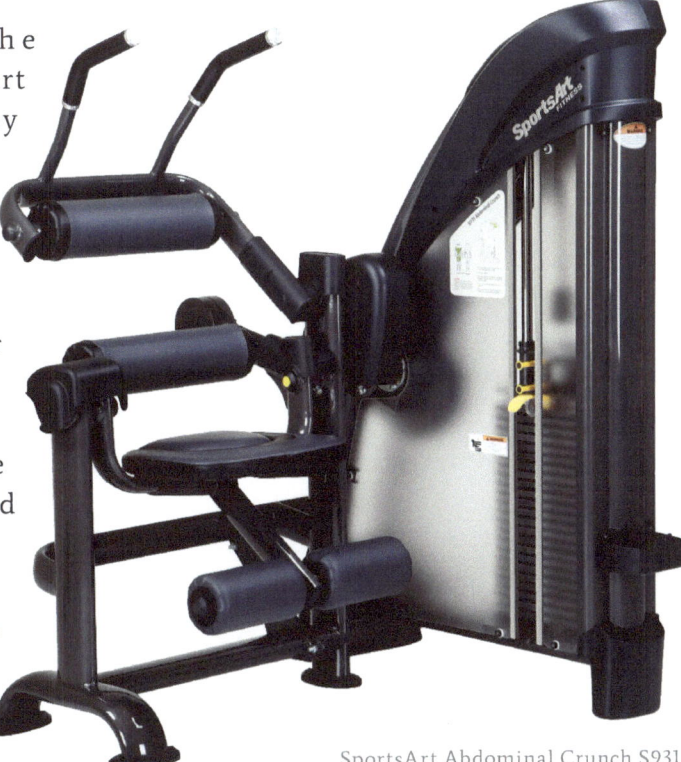

SportsArt Abdominal Crunch S931

This machine is ideal for people new to fitness, because it guarantees you're working out your abs in the right way. Without practice, it's hard to keep your feet straight and your movements smooth with traditional sit-ups and crunches. A machine will guide you through abdominal exercises correctly. Crunch machines can be as simple as a small supporting apparatus, which are less than $300, to a more complicated machine that can cost from $600 and go up from there.

Chapter 8
All-in-one Machines

There are many reasons why you might prefer an all-in-one machine. One is sheer simplicity. You'd rather avoid a set of free weights and multiple single-target machines – perfectly understandable. An all-in-one machine lets you train your whole body with ease. You might also have sensitive joints or a need to work around injuries. In this case, an all-in-one machine is a smart, safe choice. You might simply want to get the most out of limited space, or maybe you'd prefer to put a heftier, all-at-once investment into something that will give you the most bang for your buck over the long haul. Any of those reasons is good enough to give consideration to an all-in-one workout machine.

An important thing to note, however, is that most all-in-one machines don't combine strength training with cardio. You can get an all-in-one-machine strength training machine, but it is hard to find a combination cardio machine. So if you want to do cardio at home, you should consider a treadmill, elliptical, or other cardio machine to complement your strength training machine. If you prefer to breathe the fresh air and pursue jogging or swimming for your cardio, perhaps just one all-encompassing strength training machine is your best bet. Whatever your reason, there is an all-in-one machine to fit your needs and budget.

Strength Training Machines

If your goal is to build and tone muscle and increase strength, a strength training machine is ideal. Most machines use a cable and pulley system that can be adjusted for multiple exercises. They will also have a weight stack with a pin that allows you to set the proper weight level for whatever exercise you are performing. If you plan to workout with a partner or friend on a regular basis, look for a machine with two or more weight stacks so that two people can work out simultaneously. You can even find a machine with "spotting" devices to help keep you safer during high-weight workouts.

Strength training machines go up in cost and size the more adjustments and settings they have. That is, the more exercises you can perform on the machine, the more they're going to cost. Look for a machine that has at least a few leg exercises, lat-pulls, and chest and back exercises. Ideally, your machine should also include pull up bars and a dip bar. These bars will allow you to add additional exercises to your routine for variety.

If you don't want to spend thousands of dollars on a complex unit, consider purchasing a simpler one and complementing it with a set of dumbbells. If you intend to purchase a set of dumbbells, get a home gym machine with an adjustable weight bench. Between dumbbells and an all-in-one machine, you'll be able to do a hundred different exercises or more.

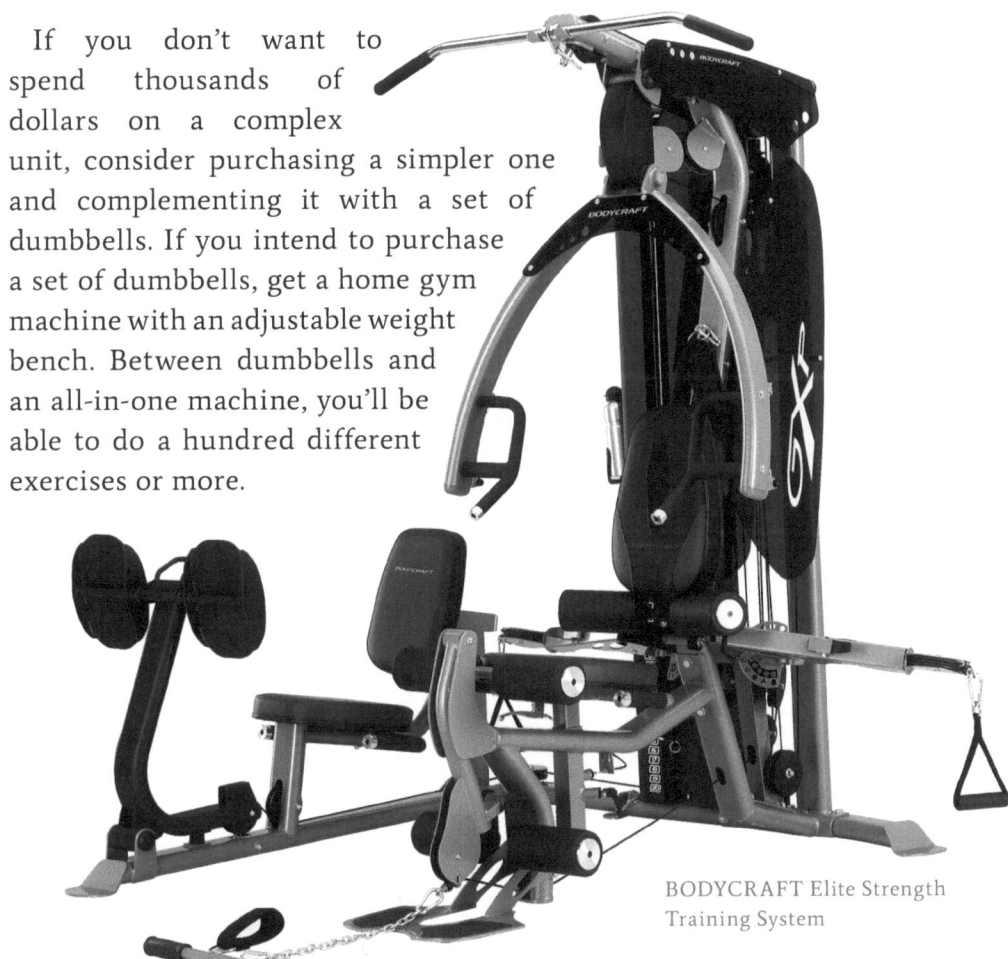

BODYCRAFT Elite Strength Training System

There are so many all-in-one strength training machines available, with new ones arriving every year, that it would be impossible to cover them all in this short book. One thing to note, however, is that all-in-one strength training machines are pricey, and for good reason: they include everything you need to get a complete workout. In lieu of buying other equipment and machines, you can simply buy one. It's convenient, but expect to pay at least $1800 for a reasonably good machine. Some machines can run well into the thousands. Your best bet is to look at "top" lists, which you can easily find online. From there, you can identify individual brand names and machines, and look up user reviews. But be fully aware that many online reviewers and publications may have an "agenda" and may well stand to profit from your purchase. Take everything you read with a grain of salt and never rely on a single review or source to come to a buying decision.

All-in-one Cardio Machines:

There aren't really any all-in-one cardio machines and that's because they're hard to design and produce. But if you're willing to put down a bit more money so as to have something a little more entertaining and versatile than a mere treadmill, try something like an adaptive motion trainer.

Adaptive motion trainers are a fairly new exercise technology and they're valuable because of their freedom of movement. Rather than traveling in the same motion or direction, you are free to move however and wherever you like. This lets you perform a range of movements to target all kinds of different muscle groups. You can do everything from short-stride rowing, to elliptical-like motions to step ups.

Adaptive motion trainers are for those really serious about fitness, or at least willing to make a serious financial investment. Since adaptive motion trainers are so new and use the latest technologies, they can get very pricey. Expect to pay a minimum of $3500 for a used machine and upwards of $9000 for a new one.

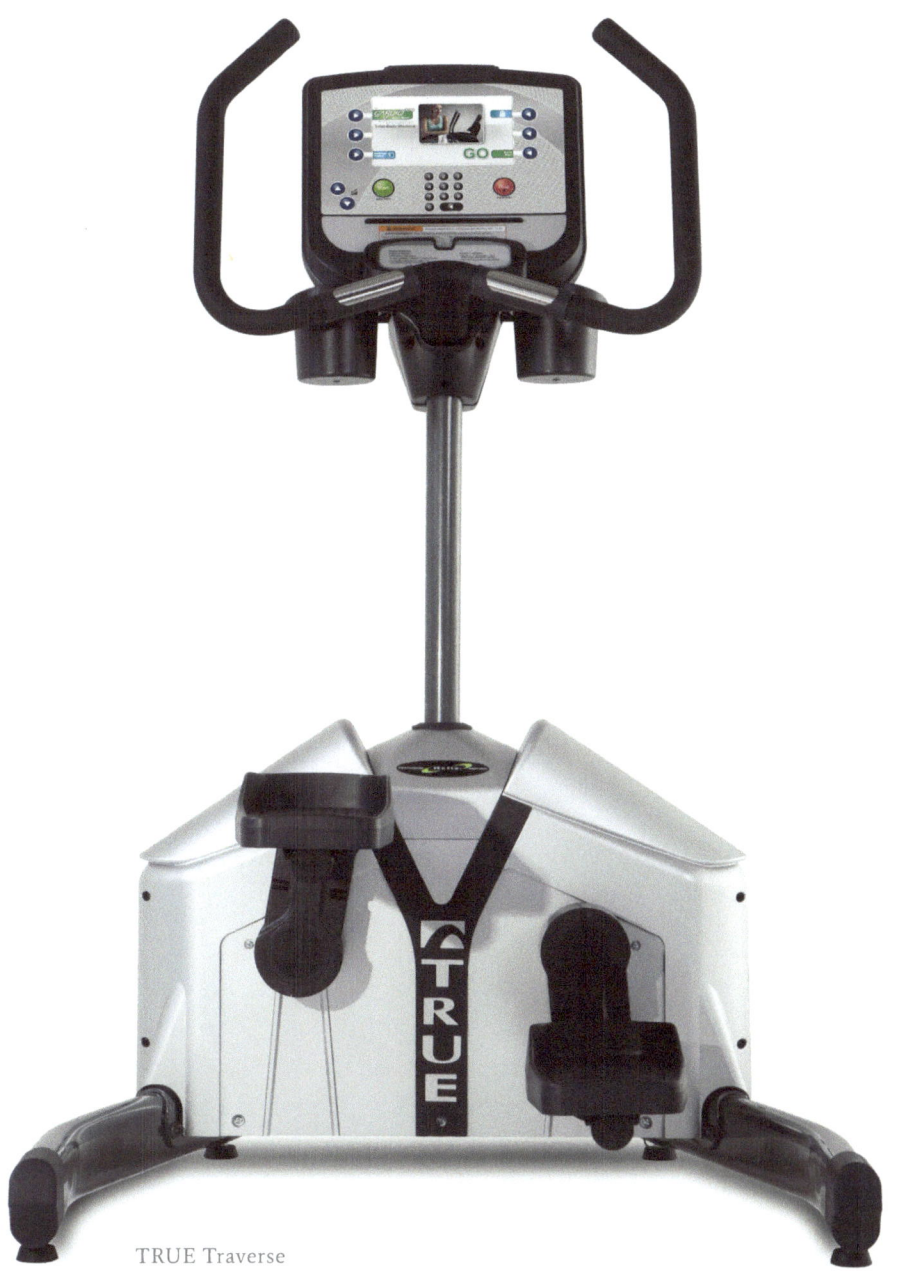

TRUE Traverse

Chapter 9
Accessories: Gloves, Belts, Wraps, Chalk, Balls, etc.

Now that you've got the basics of your home gym in place, it's time for the fun part: accessorizing. When we say "accessorizing," we mean the kinds of things you don't necessarily need, but which would be nice to have. If you have extra room in your budget or if you planned well and saved money on your other equipment and have some money leftover, indulge yourself by adding some extra items and fun things to your home gym. Not everything is simply miscellaneous – all of these items are useful, if not absolutely necessary.

Gloves: You might want to consider a pair of gloves for various exercises. If you're looking to build upper body strength and reflexes, consider investing in some boxing gloves and a punching bag. This will provide a great outlet for stress, give you an excellent upper body workout, and get your heart pumping. If you have poor grip strength, you might want to get some weight lifting gloves. These will make it easier to grip a bar or weight when your hands get sweaty. They can also be detrimental, however--you might get a false sense of your grip strength. The best method is to use them on and off, or to train your grip separately with a grip trainer. Such trainers are very cost effective. You can get a decent one for $20 to $40.

Chalk: If gloves don't sound comfortable to you, or if you want to train your grip while not suffering in the process, gym chalk is a good alternative. Just rub some on your hands for a great grip and protection against callouses. You can get a year's worth of gym chalk for $10 or less. Gym chalk is usually only used by serious weight lifters, who lift often enough that their hands actually need the added grip.

Weight Lifting Belt: Back in the old days of weight-lifting, bodybuilders used weight lifting belts. While they're largely out of fashion now, they can still be extremely beneficial. Weight lifting belts provide balance and help you get more out of your weight lifting routine. They stabilize and reduce stress on the spine. If you're thinking of getting into some serious weight lifting, a belt might be a great accessory for you. If you plan to only lift occasionally and not delve into serious levels of weight, a weight lifting belt is probably not necessary. You can find a good belt for approximately $55.

Wraps: Though exercise is meant to get you healthier, it can sometimes harm you as well, particularly if you're not careful. Regular stress caused by workouts can contribute to joint pain and injury. That's why it's important to protect your joints when you work out. Weight lifting, in particular, causes joint stress. If you already have joint problems, or have sore wrists due to excess typing or office work, it is strongly recommended that you buy wrist wraps. With wrist wraps, your wrists will be supported and stabilized during your workouts. Wraps aren't just for wrists though. You can find a wrap for any sore joint. Wraps are available for knees, elbows, and other sensitive areas, and are light and easy to put on and take off. You can also buy them in a variety of colors. Expect to pay between $20 and $60 depending on material, length, and strength.

Stability Balls: Also known as exercise balls, yoga balls, swiss balls, physioballs, etc. Stability balls are a great accessory to any home gym. They are large vinyl balls you can use to strengthen and stretch your body, improve core balance and stability, and add variety to your workout. They come in every color imaginable and they're mostly all made of the same material, so the main factor of consideration in buying should be size. You'll need to buy a ball that matches your height. If you are between 4'11" to 5'4", get a 55 cm ball. If you're between 5'4" to 5'11", you need a 65 cm ball. And if you're between 5'11" and 6'7" tall, get a 75cm or larger ball.

With a ball, even simple exercises like sit ups or push ups become more challenging and extra effective. You can even use your ball at your desk for a seat that will help maintain balance and strengthen your spine. Stability balls can benefit everyone, but they're especially useful for people who enjoy more body exercise workouts or sports, such as yoga, pilates, and gymnastics.

For maximum safety, choose an exercise ball with a high anti-burst resistance rating. We do not recommend a ball that does not list an anti-burst rating on the package. This typically means the rating is low. The strongest, safest, most burst-resistant exercise ball available is the best choice, particularly for advanced users. You'll probably pay $20 to $70 per ball, depending on size.

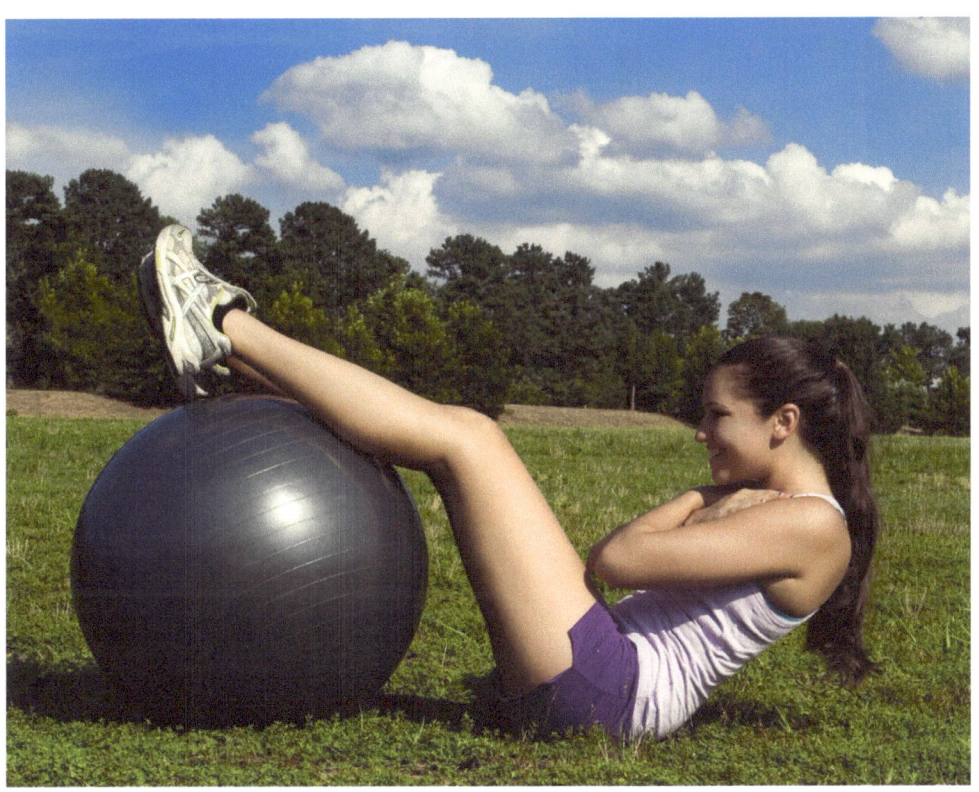

Using a stability ball in modified sit-up position, with her calves resting atop the ball, buttocks on the ground, and arms crossed over her chest.

Conclusion

For many of you, the idea of having a home gym, or some piece of home exercise equipment, has crossed your mind every New Year. But, each year, a lack of time, money, or maybe just sheer trepidation over where to start has prevented you from acting on your thoughts. Well, hopefully we've taken at least one or two of those reasons away and you're now better equipped to research, shop for, and purchase everything you need to put together your perfect home gym. You should be at ease shopping online or in a store with no fear. Armed with the knowledge you need and your carefully laid plan, no salesperson, friend, or relative will be in a position to steer you to a purchase that doesn't meet your needs. Whether you intend to have one machine or a dozen, you're now an aware and savvy consumer. Do not be deterred from your goal of better fitness and overall health.

Exercise will soon be a regular part of your day, like eating, sleeping and brushing your teeth. But as you begin your fitness journey, remember a few things. First, stay positive. Don't be too easy on yourself, but don't beat yourself up. You've already taken a positive step in reading this guide, so congratulate yourself on that. You just have to keep moving forward from here. Getting fit takes dedication and patience.

Secondly, take it one step at a time. Whatever you choose, once you have your fitness equipment purchased and installed, get into a regular and healthy routine, but know that you'll have some off days. Even the most successful athletes do. What's important is your extended effort over time – small changes will add up to a healthier you. Most importantly, get your heart pumping and have fun! Remember, you're about to be the charter member of a gym that has no dress code, no waiting line and never closes. How cool is that?

I hope you've found this guide helpful. Happy shopping, and good luck on your fitness journey!

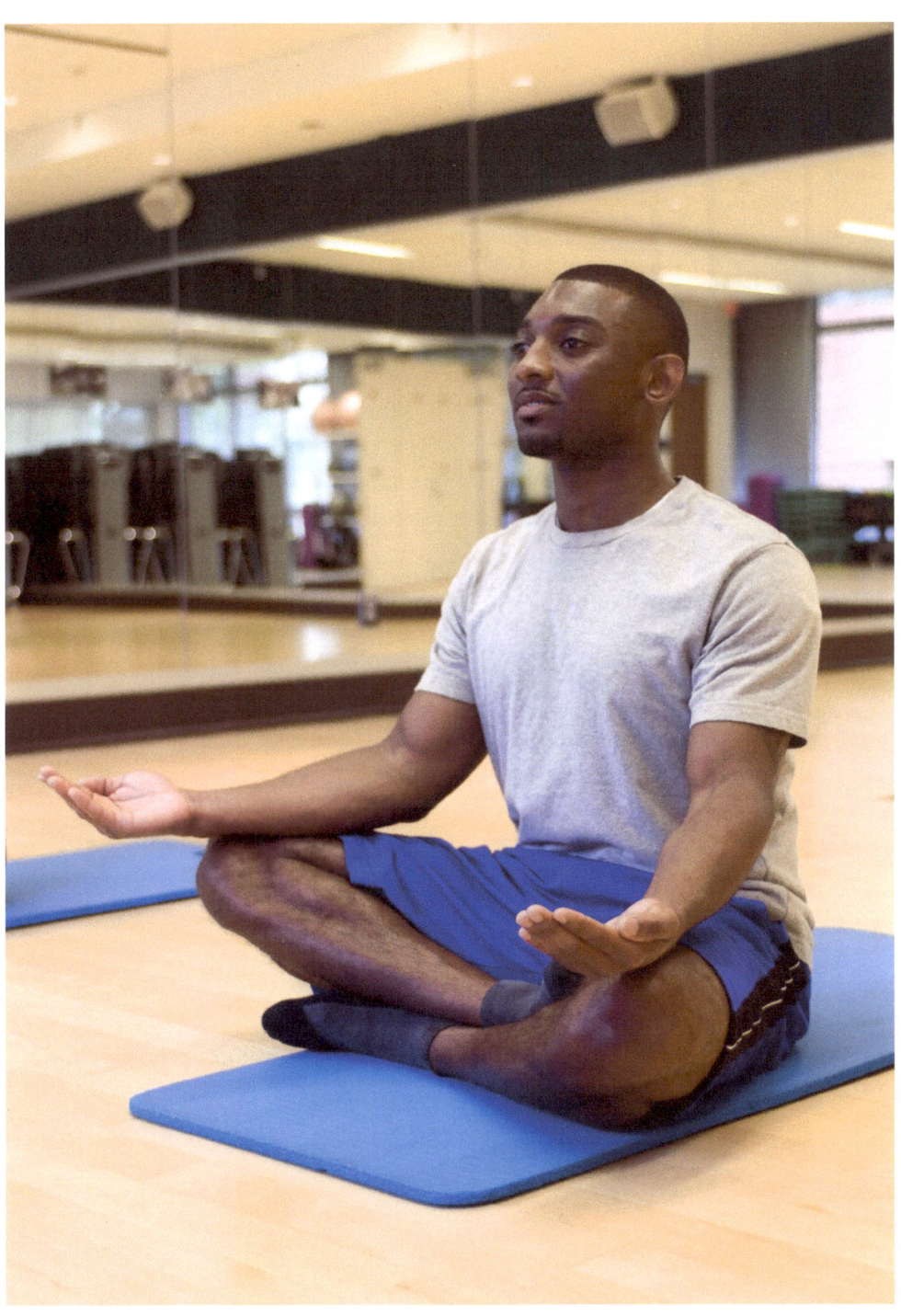

About the Author

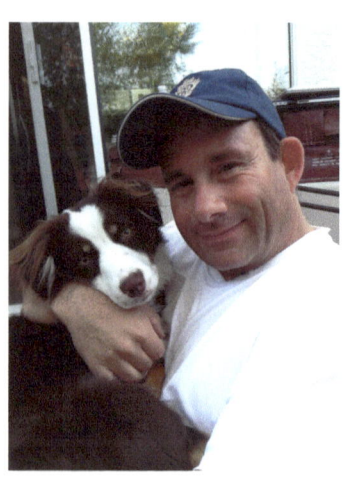

Tim Adams has been selling top-of-the-line fitness equipment in Southern California for almost 30 years. His extensive knowledge and experience, coupled with a genuine concern for his customers, allowed Tim to grow multiple fitness stores from acorns into oaks. He cultivated and catered to a loyal following of fitness professionals, coaches, trainers and instructors as well as physical therapists, nutritionists, chiropractors and sports physicians. Along the way, he also made good friends of regular, everyday customers who simply needed help selecting the right piece of fitness equipment for their homes.

After years of building businesses for others, Tim and his wife, Darci, decided to create their own retail space where they could call the shots and "do things right, every time." They conceived RX Fitness Equipment as a collaborative effort amongst health and fitness professionals with the goal of getting as many people as possible back in shape, one person at a time. And it's been a huge success.

If you've read this book, then you already know that Tim's philosophy is about much more than selling a lot of fitness equipment. It's also about encouraging those who purchase the equipment to use it, and providing them with the help and support they need to reach their weight loss and fitness goals.

RX Fitness Equipment is a major supplier of quality equipment to gyms, personal trainers, physical therapy providers, and just about every type of health and fitness facility that you can imagine. But, Tim is also here to serve the needs of those in search of the single perfect piece of home exercise equipment, or an entire home gym. Don't hesitate to take advantage of his expertise.

Tim can be reached at T.Adams@rxfitnessequipment.com or by calling the store in Thousand Oaks, California at (805) 409-8600.

RX Fitness Equipment
2388-2 Thousand Oaks Blvd
Thousand Oaks, California 91362
805.409.8600
www.RXFitnessEquipment.com

Acknowledgments

We would like to express our sincere thanks to the following manufacturers for allowing the use of their product photos to illustrate this book.

Bodycraft

Bodyguard Fitness

Spirit Fitness

SportsArt

TRUE Fitness

Thanks to the many talents and "sets of eyes" involved in creating and editing this book, especially **Darci Adams**. Your help and support was invaluable.

Graphic Design and Layout
Carl Bluemel
www.BluemelCreative.com

Editing and Publication
Social Media Toolworks
www.SocialMediaToolworks.com

The information provided in this book is for general research purposes only. It is not intended as, and does not constitute, professional advice. We do not recommend any particular brand or type of equipment, nor do we advise embarking on any routine of strenuous exercise without first consulting your physician to determine that you are healthy enough to participate in an exercise program.

www.ingramcontent.com/pod-product-compliance
Lightning Source LLC
Chambersburg PA
CBHW040311010626
45792CB00022B/171